Acupuncture and Cellular Molecule Biology

—The Theoretical Base of Chinese Medicine

Akupunktur und Zellen Molekule Biologie

—Die Theoretischen Basis der Chinesische Medizin

针灸 与 细胞分子生物学

— 兼论中医的理论基础

CONTENT

INTRODUCTION

(ABSTRACT)

The basic theory of the West Medicine is anatomy, the fundamental principle of the Chinese Medicine is meridian. Before 5000 years the great talents of past China discovered the phenomena of meridian in human body, and used herbs and acupuncture to cure illness successfully, which guaranteed the multiplication of Chinese nation and the development of Chinese culture uninterrupted.

The author of this book began to contact Traditional Chinese Medicine (TCM) in 1988 and was interested in the theory of meridian. Under the inspiration of "Unification between Heaven and human" of Daoism, through more than 10 years' thinking and recent 10 years of research and exploration, the author realized gradually, **"the phenomenon of meridian is the result of interaction between the activity of electro-physiology (mainly of heart and brain) of human body and the physical field of solar-earth (mainly geo-magnet field), the interaction induces the Lorentz -Force, and subsonic vibration and then, produces bio-wave (acoustic wave) conducting and spreading in all the human body. Meridian is the tunnel of the bio-wave of human body. The phenomenon of meridian is an effect of bio-physical field. For researching meridian it's no meaning to look for the anatomy structure of meridian in human body. Every organ, every tissue and every cell all are the carriers of meridian".**

Author's research for meridian is based on the Modern Cell Molecular Biology and the Modern Solar-Earth Physics, as well as the interdisciplinary and extension of the above two grand scientific subjects. Thus, the bio-physical model and bio-mathematical model of the Modern Meridian Science have been established. The author has calculated the phase velocity, amplitude, frequency and energy of the bio-wave in meridian. This wave is a **Transversal Wave** which vibration direction is vertical with the direction of the wave's conducting direction along the meridian but **Longitudinal Wave.**

Just by the action of conduction of bio-wave in the body, all the cells of the body are in the situation of vibration. This vibration guarantees the fluidity and mobility of membrane which is composed by lipid double-layers and with liquid-crystal structure; thereby realizes the exchange of substances, energy and information between membrane and micro-circulation, endocrine and nerve system. The action of bio-wave also guarantees the synthesis and secretion of protein, enzyme, fat and carbohydrate in plasma and inner membrane, together with the support of cytoskeleton and exchange of energy (ATP). At least bio-wave guarantees the normal storage, replication, transcription of genetic materials, cell's division and hyperplasia. For this discovery author advance a new scientific subject — **"The Dynamics of Wave to Cell"** which is a new subject researching of the interaction between bio-wave and cell specially.

The author discovered that except sunshine, air and water, the geo-magnetic field is the fourth guarantee for human's life. The oldest geo-magnetic rock has the age of 3.5 billion years and the oldest microbe also has 3.5 billion years age, this fact illustrates geo-magnetic field is how important for the life in the earth.

The theory of bio-wave could completely explain the follows experimental and clinic phenomena, such as: low electro resistance and low acoustic resistance along meridian, flowing trace of labelled atoms is within meridian lines, Narcotisation and Analgesia by Acupuncture. This theory can explain why the lipid double-layers of membrane can move with more than 6 kinds patterns; the transport of protein, enzyme and other materials can pass through the membrane, etc. It can also explain the discoveries by the ancient Chinese doctors, such as: "Meridian moving in the surface of body in the day time and in the inner body in the night" <Nan Jing 难经>; "Phlegm resistances the motion of meridian" <Huang Di Nei Jing 黄帝内经>, etc.

<Huang Di Nei Jing (Classic Internal Medicine of Yellow Emperor)> written before 2500 years said, "Meridian could decide life or dead, treat and cure for hundred kinds of illness and regulate deficiency and excess of physique of human. Meridian must be unobstructed." In this book the author gives the new definition for "Qi 气 " and " Xue (Blood) 血 " in TCM. **"Qi" is the propagation of bio-wave with audio frequency all over the human body; "Xue" is the blood circulation and micro-circulation system.** The regulation and balance of "Qi" and "Xue" have been paid attention by TCM which maintains regular metabolism, enhances immunity and self reha-capability. This book **collects and presents** much more cases for curing hepatic diseases (especially for hepatocarcinoma and cirrhosis) with great length. These recipes of the cases were adopted by the ancient and modern famous experts of TCM within 2000 years period. The basic theory of their treatments is "Yin-Yang" theory and "Wu Xing" principles. The experts laid stress on the regulation of "Qi" and "Xue" to enhance self-immunity of patients, but pay attention to virus and bacteria, operation and transplantation.

In chapter 2 of The Therapy by Acupuncture, author puts forward the theory of "Interference Wave" in meridian. When needles prick into body, the bio-wave is synthesized and transformed into the **Standing Wave** with greater amplitude and energy, which enhance the fluidity and mobility of membrane, especially the enrichment and oscillation of Ca^{++} promote the metabolism and the exchange of substance, energy and information between cell and micro-circulation, security, lymph as well as nerve-system. This theory could explain all the follows questions: Why acupuncture can cure illness? Why the stimulation of acupuncture can be conducted with two opposite direction? (Nerve system is single directive conduction.) Why could two opposite diseases be cured by same acu-points by acupuncture? e.g. when pricking one point (e.g. PC 6 or LI 11), acupuncture can either decrease blood pressure for hypertension patient, or increase blood pressure for hypotension patient.

In chapter 3 author put forward the theory of "Synapse Block" of nerve system, which can explain the principle of acupuncture-analgesia and -anaesthesia by nerve molecular biology. The bigger amplitude interference bio-wave makes the K^+ across the cell membrane outside, and the rest potential will be higher, this "Hyperpolarization Phenomena" makes the threshold actional potential of depolarization higher. At same time, under the very strong stimulation of Acupuncture Manuela, the oscillation of Ca^{++} by standing wave happened and only in original place, the reflux of Ca^{++} entering into C nerve ending becomes more difficult and the cytocest in pre-synapes could not be transported to the membrane, which prevents the releasing of P material, glutamic acid and other more than 50 kinds of transmitters into the cleft between pre- and post-synapes. Thus, post-synaps cannot appear depolarization, acupuncture makes the time of action potential of DRG (dorsal Root Ganglion) shorter, decreases neuro electric current transmitting up and realizes the aim of analgesia and anaesthesia.

In chapter 4 Author analysed the two characters of cancer cells (anoxybiontic and low electro-potential voltage of membrane), revealed the principle of therapy of Qigong. The special effect of "Guo Lin Qigong" for curing cancer was described with 2 typical cases.

In this book author introduced the effect of **Chinese herbs therapy** of hepatopathies with more pages, including rescuing for serious hepatic coma and hepatocarcinoma, collected the success cases of treatment for hepatoparthy by the past and modern Chinese famous TCM experts, involving for the illness of acute and chronic hepatitis, hepatocirrhose, ascites due to cirrhose, hepatocarcinoma and hepatic coma. In this book about 11 cases, 23 recipes of herbs and 12 "plus or minus" recipes were introduced. The **"differentiation principle"** were emphasised and analysed in detail in all the cases.

The author introduced about more than 10 kinds of Chinese herbs which are always used to therapy hepatopathy. The names of herbs are written by the languages of Chinese, PINYIN, English, Germany and Latin respectively and with colour pictures. The function of the herbs is described with different effect for anti-ictero, clearing heat, eliminating damp, tonic of Qi, cooling blood, tonic of blood, activating blood, breaking block, nourishing liver, tonic of spleen, tonic of kidney, etc.

With the theory of "Bio-Wave of Meridian" put forward by author and the foundation of cellular molecular biology, the theory base of therapy by herbs were illustrated in chapter 7.

In chapter 8 author collected 9 kinds of adopting Acu-Points recipes for therapy of icterohepatitis, chronic hepatitis and hepatocirrhose.

In recent years there are some gratifying news to prove the existence of bio-wave in meridian and its function to the human's life (see Chapter 1).

I have put forward the concept of "Bio-Wave", "Standing Wave, "Important Function of Ca^{++}" and "Synaps Block", etc. but the referential research & experiment are only at beginning progress now. Author warmly welcomes the criticism and supervision of scholars in all circles. It is a huge challenge to confirm the existence of bio-wave in human body and its function for the physiology and pathology, specially the relation between acupuncture and cell molecular biology as well as nerve molecular biology.

Author

Winter 2018

Left bank of Rhein

1. The Meridian Phenomena

1.1 Meridian (Jing Luo) is the tunnel of Biological-Wave over all the Human Body

In Chinese medicine, the Meridian (Jing Luo 经络) including14 Jing Mai (经脉 meridian lines) and the Luo Mai (络脉 the innumerable branches of Jing Mai) are arranged over all the **living man's body**. The theory of Meridian is considered to be the guiding principle of the physiology and pathology of human body in TCM.

It's a vain attempt to look for the anatomy structure of meridian. The phenomena of meridian exist in every organ and tissue, as well as in every cell. We would say total body is the anatomy structure of meridian.

Jing Luo isn't an anatomy tissue. Jing Luo is the tunnels of the biological wave. This wave is produced by the interaction between the magnetic field of solar-earth and the electro-physiological phenomena of heart and brain of human body.

《Hunag Di Nei Jing 黄帝内经》 was the authority and classic lexicon of Chinese medicine, which was written by dialogue between Huang Di and Dr. Qi Bo before 2500 years (Fig. 1) which emphasized: "Jing Luo, decides man is living or death, treatments every kinds of illness, regulates Yin and Yang." The birth, oldness, illness and death all are regulated and decided by meridian situation. If meridian floats unobstructed, Qi and blood are abundant and full, healthy Qi is ascending and pathogenic Qi can not disturb the body, men will be healthy, anti-illness and longevity.

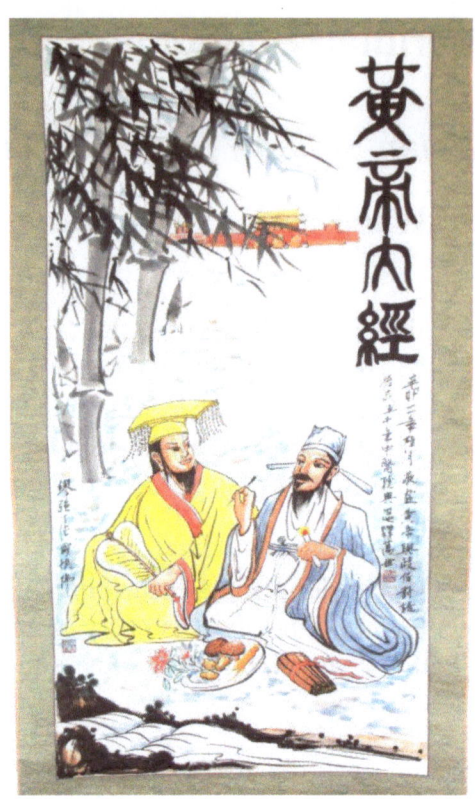

Fig. 1 《Huang Di Nei Jing》 Dialog between Yellow Emperor with Dr. Qi Bo

Oppositely if the meridian blocked, Qi and Blood stopped and stasis, the metabolism is declined, the substances exchange between micro-circulation and membranes of cells is failed, the inter-change of information and transmitters between the central nerve and lymph systems with every organ will be blocked, and different illness will be appeared.

The block of meridian is due to the obstruction of bio-wave in human body.

The theory of "Bio-Wave of Jing Luo" put forward and discovered by author is composed by following parts:

14

1.2 Meridian Phenomena is the Effect of Field

Meridian phenomenon is a bio-physical "Field Effect", which has no relation with "Anatomy Structure".

1. 3 "Cosmos-Physiology"

Put forward and established by author is a new scientific subject which researches the interaction between the physical phenomena of cosmos (inclusive solar and earth) and the physiological activities of human body when lay up the person in the surface of the earth (Fig.2). "Cosmos-Physiology" is different with the subjects of "Astrobiology", "Cosmic-Physiology" and "cosmobiology", which lay up the people into space but in earth surface.

The main difference between "Cosmos-Physiology" and "Physiology" is "Cosmos-Physiology" takes thinking of the function of physical field of Solar-earth (mainly the geo-magnetic field) to the physiology of human body, which can explore the meridian theory of TCM. At same time this could explain much more physiological and pathological questions that have not been understood and known until now and will develop the life science (see Fig.3 "Qi, Meridian").

1.4 The Lorentz Force and the Production of Bio-Wave with Quantum Theory

Since we have not found the anatomy tissue of meridian until now, according the theory of quantum, every thing has the dual character (article and wave), I try to look for the existence of wave for meridian.

The Meridian Phenomena is the result of the interaction between **Electro-Physiology Phenomena** of human body (Central Nervous and autonomic nerve System, Fig.4, as well as electro-cardiology system, Fig.5,) and the Solar-Earth Physics Field（mainly is **geo-magnetic field**, Fig. 6). This interaction produces the cyclical **Lorentz Force** (Fig.7) acting on the tissues with **subsonnic frequency** (Fig. 8). In the **"meridian model of bio-physics"**, this cyclical force produces a **"Forced Vibration"** with **sonic frequency** (Fig. 9) in the heart and nerve systems' tissues structure, and then the vibration induces bio-wave transmitting into the total body (Fig. 10). The synthetic waves will conduct along some main tunnels (Jing Luo) and then into the nets of organs and total cells of the body, which make all the cells in a situation of micro-vibration with **sonic spectrum of frequency**. The main tunnels are the 14 meridian lines of "Jing Luo 经络". The nets of "Luo Mai 络脉" is composed by "Luo Zi 络子" and "Luo Sun 络孙".

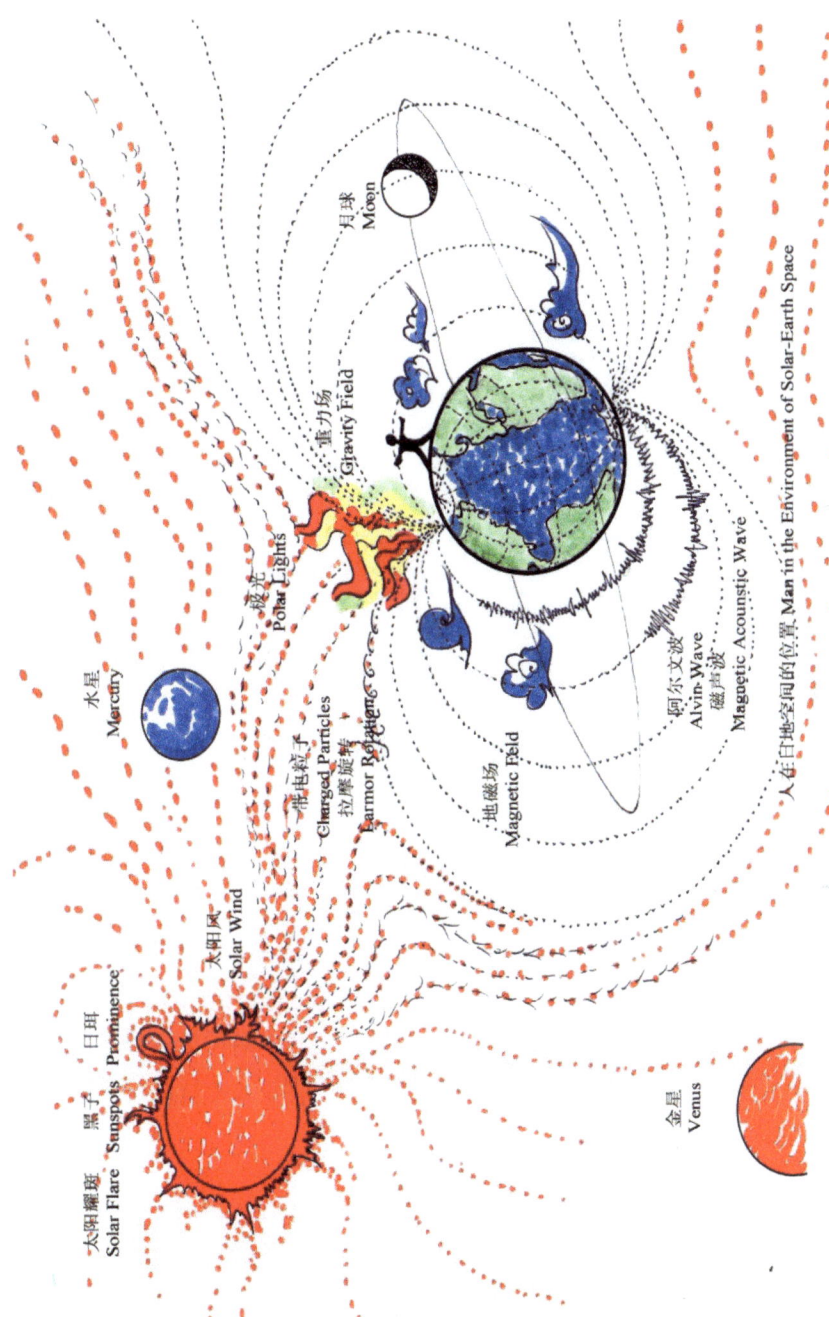

Fig. 2 The Position of Man in the Space of Solar-Earth

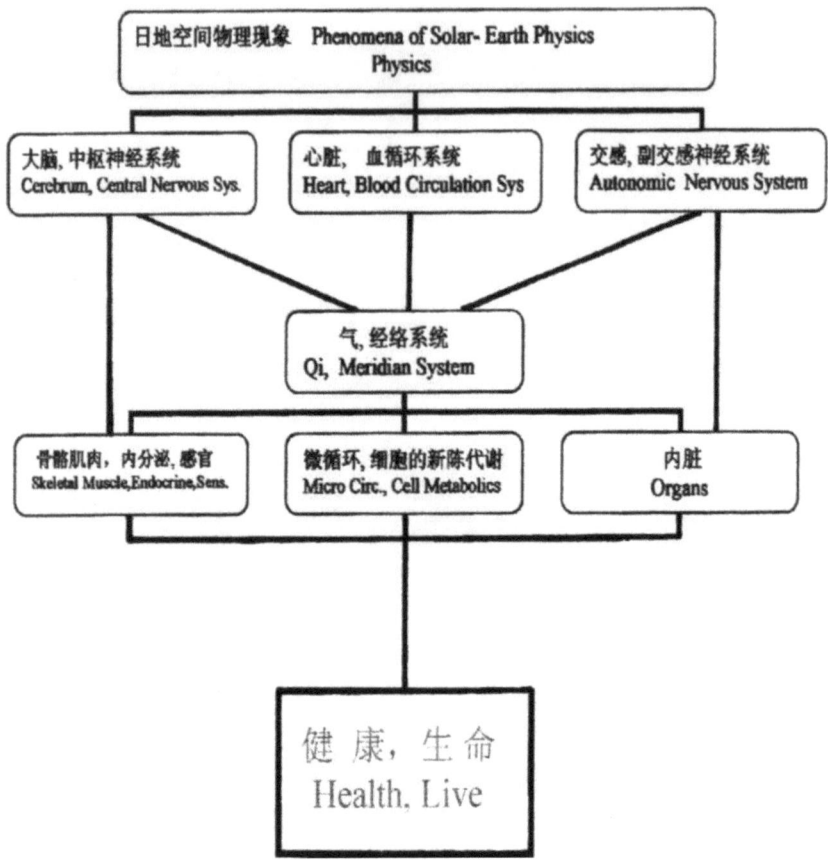

Fig. 3 The Interaction between Geo-Magnetic Field and Three Electro-Physiology. The Production of Meridian System Meridian

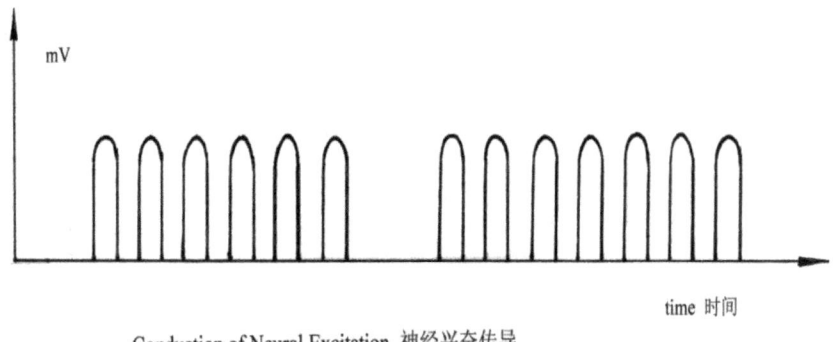

Conduction of Neural Excitation 神经兴奋传导
Frequency 20-50 Hz

Fig. 4 Neural excitation of cerebrate central nervous

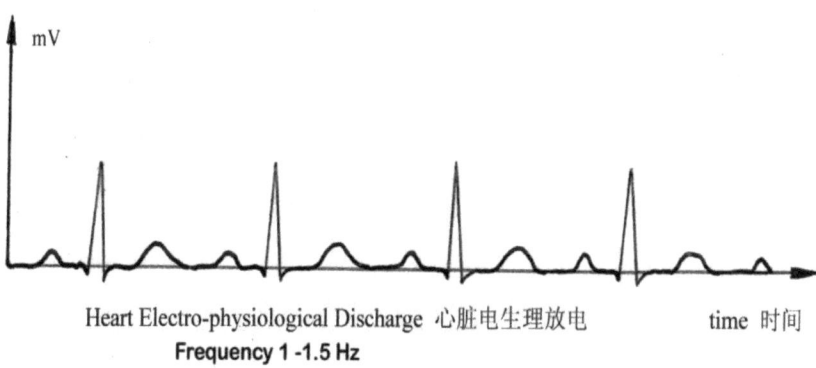

Heart Electro-physiological Discharge 心脏电生理放电
Frequency 1 -1.5 Hz

Fig. 5 Discharge of heart electro-physiology

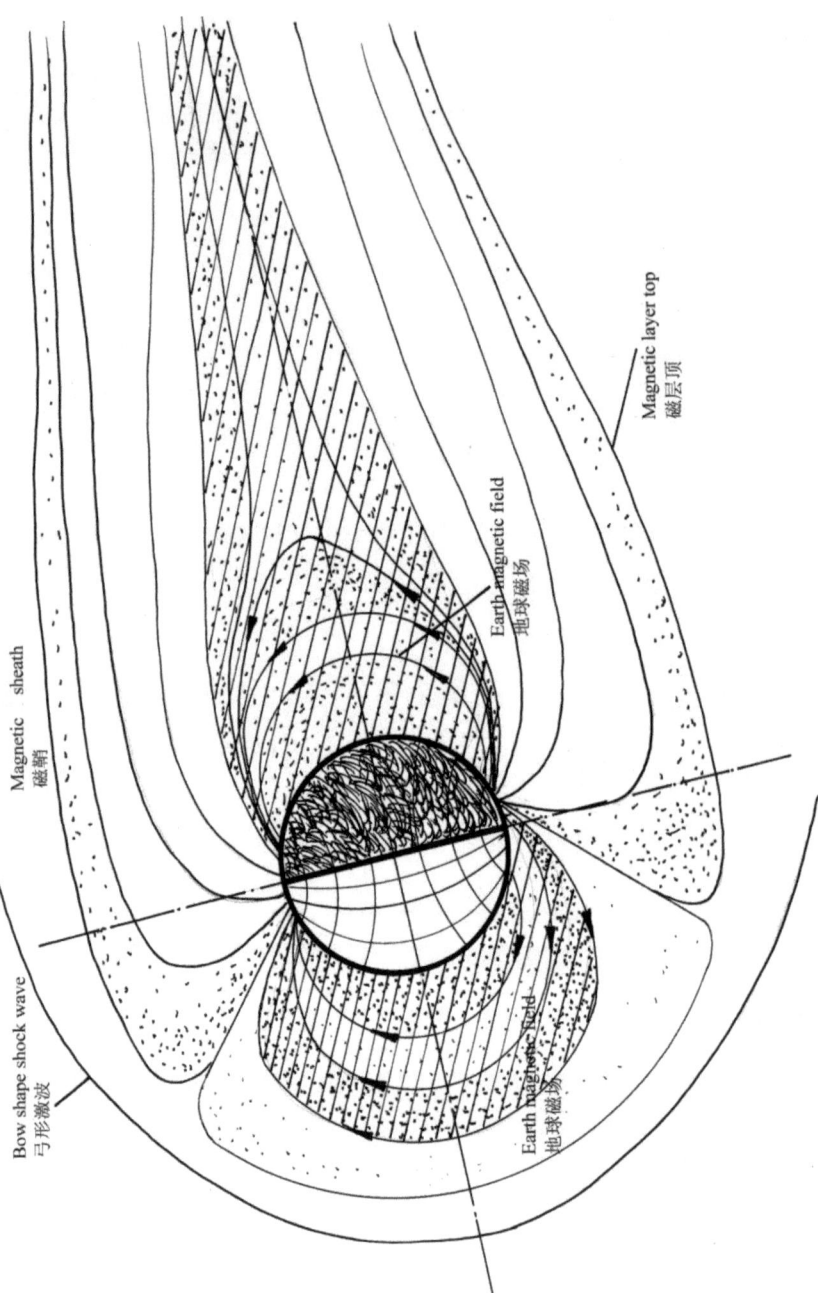

The follows are the bio-physical deducing process and referential calculation of production of the bio-wave in human body in detail:

The cyclical force with subsonic frequency is the Lorentz Force F (Fig. 7) which is produced by the interaction between electr-physiological current of the above two systems of the body and the geo-magnetic fields (and sometimes the magnetic field of the plasma of solar wind).

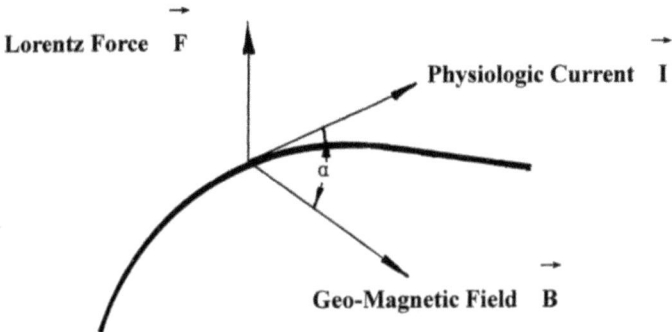

Fig.7 Lorentz Force produced by the interaction between Physiologic Current and Geo-Magnet Field

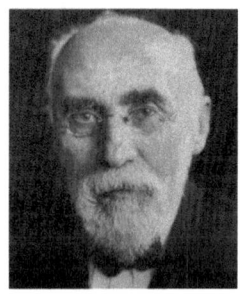

**Fig. 7a Hendrik Antoon Lorentz
1853- 1928 Niederland
1905 Nobel Prize owner**

$$\vec{F} = q\,\vec{v}\,x\,\vec{B}$$

q is the electric charge of action of electro-physiology of human body

v is the velocity of moving electric charge

$\overrightarrow{\textbf{B}}$ is the geo-magnetic field intensity

In calculation of the electro-dynamical force, **q x V** can also be replaced by electro-physiological currents **I**. The currents include nerve electric current and cardio electric current **I**.

$$\overrightarrow{F} = \int_L d \ \overrightarrow{F} = \int_L \overrightarrow{I} \ d \ \overrightarrow{1} \ x \ \overrightarrow{B}$$

When **L** is a straight line

$$F = I \ L \ B \ \sin \alpha$$

α is the angel between current I and magnetic field B. L is length of electric carries.

These electric carriers include: (1) Cardiac-Electro system: sinuatrial node, internode, A-V node, His bundle, R. and L. Bundle and Purkinje's fiber nets. (2) Center nerve system: serebrum (12 pairs), cerebellum, brain stem, spinalnerve (31 pairs), isodentritic neurons, nerve ending. (3) Autonomic nerve system: (3.1) sympathetic nerve system: brain, nerves III, VII, IX, II, pelvic splanchnic nerves, organ nerves. (3.2) parasympathetic nerve system: brain stem, T1-T12, L1, L2, organ nerves.

The Lorentz cyclical force $F = f \cos(\omega't)$, Frequency ω' is in the subsonic spectrum, which is closed with heart impulse and neural excitation (1–100HZ). Force **F** induces the forced damping oscillation on the tissues carried with electric currents.

The follows are the equation of the **forced damping oscillation**:

$$\left(\frac{dx}{dt}\right)^2 + 2\beta \frac{dx}{dt} + \omega_0 X = F = f \cos(\omega' t)$$

the solutions:

$$\tan \varphi' = \frac{2\beta\omega'}{\omega'^2 - \omega_0^2}, \quad A' = \frac{F/m}{\sqrt{(\omega'^2 - \omega_0^2)^2 + 4\beta^2\omega'^2}}$$

The intrinsic frequency ω0 of human body (organ, bone, muscle, tissue etc.) is in audio spectrum, about 100-10000 HZ. That means the frequency ω' of forced force F is greatly smaller than the intrinsic frequency ω0, i.e. ω' << ω₀ .

$$\omega' << \omega_0, A' = \frac{F/m}{\omega^2} = \frac{F}{k}$$

The vibration amplitude A' hasn't relation with the frequency of the forced force ω' nearly, as result of calculation, the amplitude of tissues is about in scale of nanos. This tissue's vibration will induces the conduction of bio-wave in the body (Fig.11).

Due to the direction of vibration is vertical with meridian, the bio-wave is a **transversal wave** (Fig.12). Of course some small longitudinal wave would be appeared also. The energy intensity of the bio-wave in 14 meridians is higher (about 0.1 erg) than other parts of the body. The velocity of the wave along meridian $\mathbf{v} = (\mathbf{G}/\rho)^{\frac{1}{2}}$ is about 1000 – 1600 m/s(G shear model, ρ density). It must be emphasized that the velocity of central nerve's current is 120m/sec maximum, only one tenth of the bio-wave. The second difference between nerve and meridian is conducting of meridian is double directions but nerve is single direction.

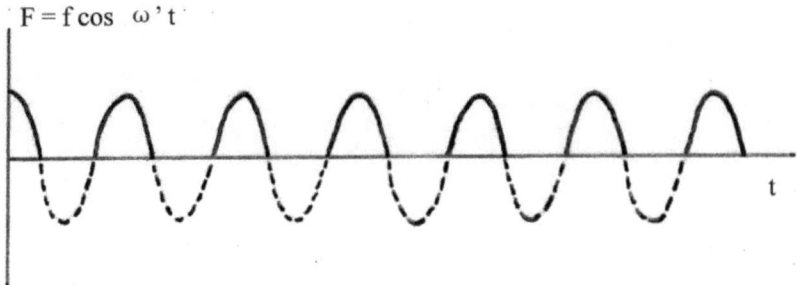

Frequency: 1-50Hz

Fig.8 Lorenz Force with Subsonic vibration spectrum in human tissue

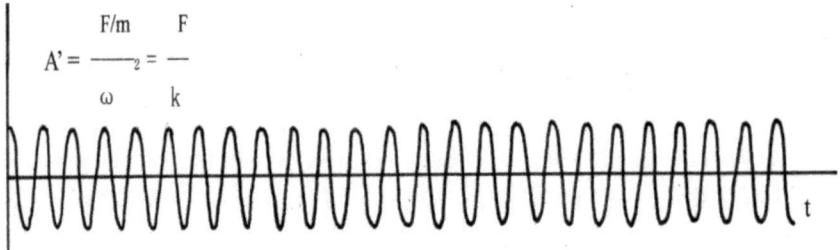

Frequency 100 – 10000 Hz

Fig. 9 Vibration of Bio-wave frequency in tissue

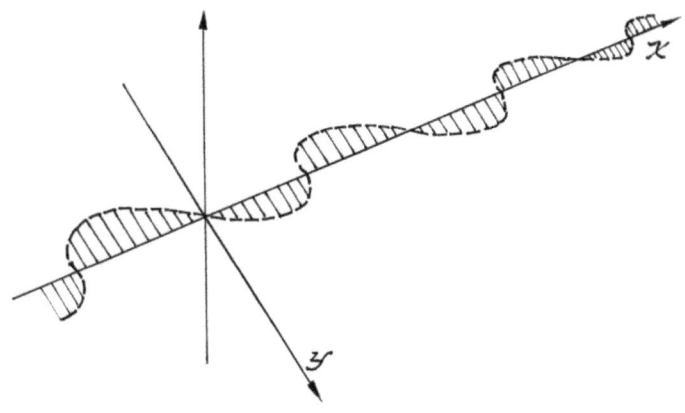

Fig. 10 The Transversal Wave conducts in Meridian Tunnel

Velocity of wave: 1000 – 1600 m/sec

X Coordinate axis is along Meridian Line, Y Axis is Vibration Direction

---

Valley Effect of Meridian

The theory of bio-wave could explain the conclusion in 《Huang Di Nei Jing》 that "meridian exist between neighbor muscles and neighbor bones". For explaining this point of view author put forward the theory of "Valley Effect of Meridian". It's well Known that the sound intensity in wave guide (such as music tube) or in valley is greatly bigger than in diffuse radiation. The spread of bio-wave in human body is same. Generally speaking most of meridian exist between muscles and between bones, for example between tibia and fibula, between ulna and radius, in the middle of gastrocnemius, etc. These position all are in low-lying area. In these areas the intensity of bio-wave is stronger, the valley effect is formed.

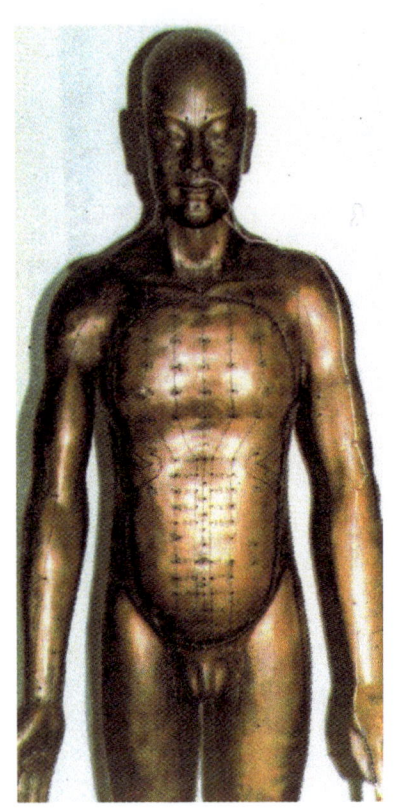 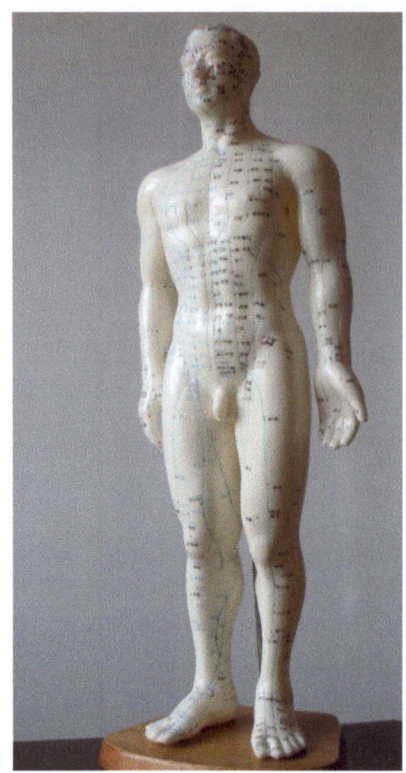

Ancient Bronze Acupuncture Figure

A.D. 1027 Song Dynasty

Fig. 11   The 14 Meridian of Human Body

1.5. Dynamic of Wave to Cell

The modern Cell Molecular Biology appointed the normal cells' membrane are in the situation of liquid crystals, all the material, energy and signals transfer between cell and outside should be in the condition of movement and fluidity of lipid bilayer structure. These movements and fluidity of membrane have more than 6 different forms (swing left and right, movement up and down, rotation of double layer, rotation of single layer, movement of

26

district, rolling up and down, etc. Fig. 12). The existence of bio-wave realizes the full movement and fluidity of membrane and supply the energy to the operation of Na^+—K^+ pump and maintain transmembrane potential (-90mV, Fig.13). Thereby realizes the exchange of substances, energy and information between cell and micro-circulation, endocrine and nerve system. The action of bio-wave also guarantees the synthesis and secretion of protein, enzyme, fat and carbohydrate in plasma and inner membrane, together with the support of cytoskeleton and exchange of energy (ATP). At least bio-wave guarantees the normal storage, replication, transcription of genetic materials, cell's division and hyperplasia. Even if the meridian activity is an energy dissipating and entropy increasing (dQ/T>0) system, it guarantees the life and health of people.

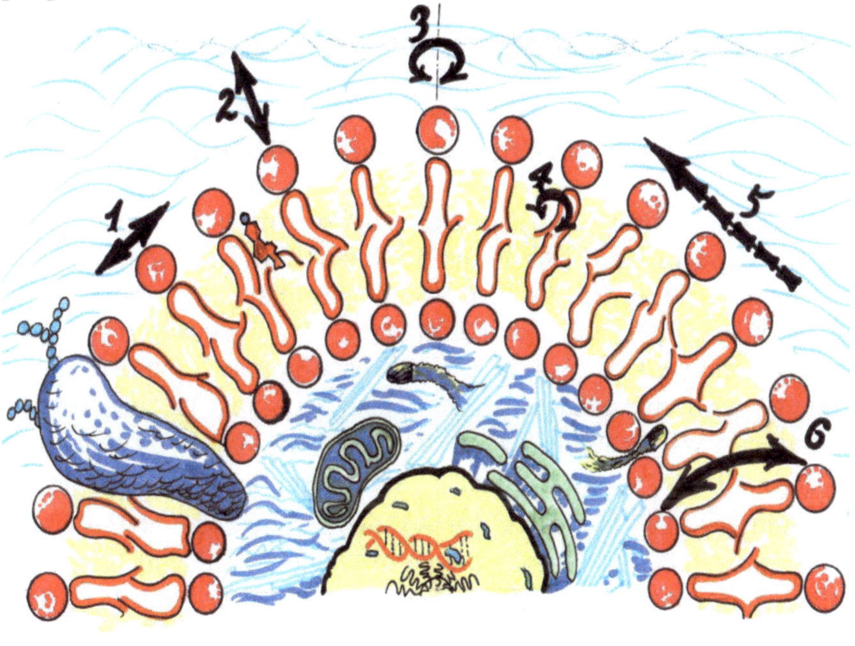

细胞膜双脂分子层的6种震动和流动状态 6 Kinds of Vibration and Fluid Situation for the Double Molecular of Cell Membrane

Fig. 12 Six Kinds of movement and Fluid Situation for Lipid Bilayer of Cell Membrane

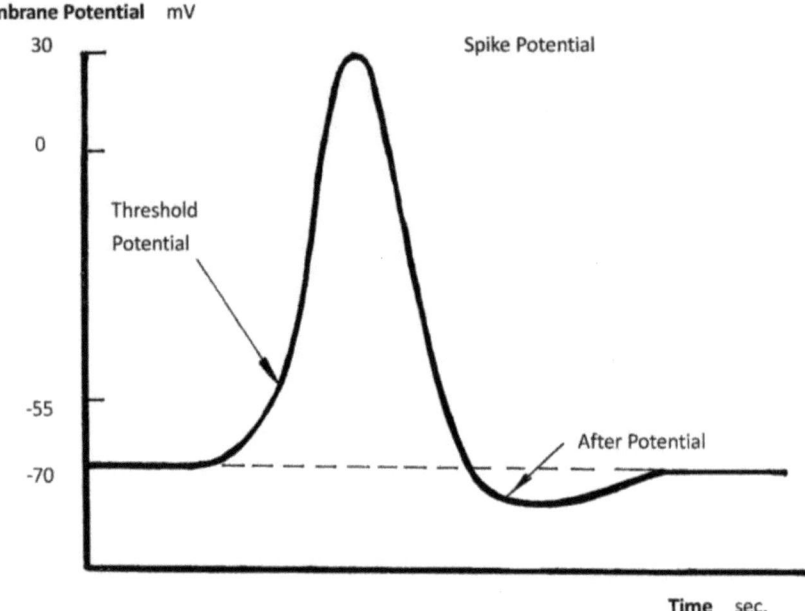

Fig.13 The Transmembrane Potential

The Fundamentals of "Bio-Wave in Meridian" could explain all the experimental phenomena of meridian and acupuncture in the last 50 years, such as, along meridian there are follows phenomena: low electric resistance, low acoustic resistance, centralization of K^+, Na^+, Ca^{++} in acu-points, labelled atoms fluidity with meridian lines, and also can answer the follows questions: Why might person be ill? Why could acupuncture therapy illness? （in Chapter 5 author supply the principle of "Standing Wave" to explain the reason） Why acupuncture could have the effects of double direction's regulation? For example, when stimulating the points of Nei Guan (PC 6) or Shen Men (HT 7), it either cures hypertension, or increases blood pressure for hypotension; it can either inhibit tachycardia or cures bradycardia. Why Qigong can therapy cancers? Etc.

The theory of bio-wave could also interpret referential classical principles of 《Huang Di Nei Jing》, such as "meridian can decide life or death, can cure hundred illness, and regulate Yin and Yang".

28

The follows important experiments of Cell Molecular Biology proved the validity and correction for the scientific judgement of bio-wave in meridian.

(1) Fig. 14 shows after the action of subsonic wave to the epithelial cells in vascular wall the obvious change of membrane, plasma and nuclear of cells, specially the microfilaments, microtubules in plasma. (Prof. GUO Yao, REN Dong Qing 《The Base and Experiment Methods of Micro Circulation, Feb. 2005》.

(2) China-Japan friendship hospital (Beijing, China) discovered in clinic that there is a micro-vibration along meridian line. The energy is about 10% of the heart pulse. This vibration was detected with the instrument of precise sensors which was made by Yan Huang JingLuo Research Center and Chinese TCM Academy.

(3) Prof. XU Qi Wang (Chongqing 3rd Military Medical University) discovers "One kind of Rate-Movement of Bio-Wave which controls the health of human" 《Dialog between Modulator of Bio-Wave and Bio-Wave》 ("People's Daily" 20, 07, 2011)

(4) Dr. Geng Li etc. 14 scientists in the acupuncture experiment of magnetic resonance elastography found Ca^{++} activated and transvers acoustic wave along meridian appears at same time. Springer Published online 2011 Jul. 28. Doi: 10.1007/s00424-011-0993-7.

(5) Dr. CHEN Wei Ju irradiated to human retina with laser, and recorded total process with high-speed camera. The experimental results not only show the saccade and vergence of the eye, but also recorded numerous moving and glistenning speckles, such as the sky is twinkling with stars. Until now this phenomena could not be explained, from my point of view, this is due to the vibration of liquid crystal structure of retina is caused by bio-wave, and then the dynamic laser interference image happened. (<Laser Speckle Dynamic Analysis of Human Retina>, The Abstract of Annual Report of Chinese Scholars Association in Germany 2012, Frankfurt)

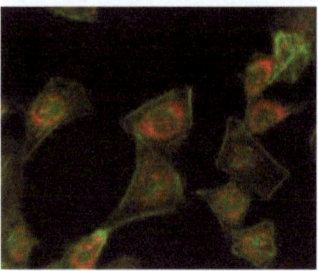

1. Before the emission of subsonic, there are only a few amount of F- actin. Staining nuclear is red colour, staining F-Actin and membrane are green.colour.

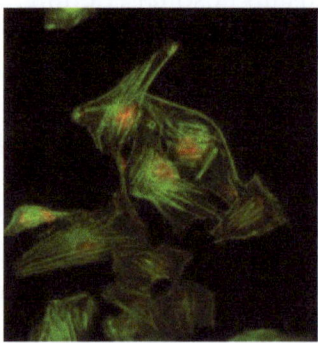

2. After one time of action of subsonic wave (160db 2h), F-actin in plasma became longer, thicker and more along the longitude axis, the fluorescence became stronger. Membrane also thicker.

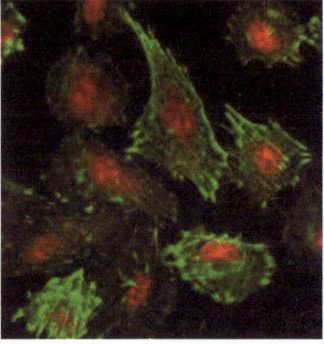

3. After 3 times action of subsonic wave, more nuclears became circular form, membrane was discontinuity, F-Actin became much more thicker, some of them were granular and nets structure with radiation and un-regular forms. Membranes are with non-continuity fluorescence lines.

Fig.14 After subsonic wave's emission to the epithelial cells of vascular wall (16Hz, 160dB, 2 h), the membrane,

F-actin, microtube in plasma and nuclear have been changed obviously

In 1988 author organized and jointed the design, manufacture of instruments of the bionic subsonic generator and meridian tester. From 2008 under the simulation of micro-wave, infrared, subsonic, acoustic etc. cosmos physical fields, author has researched their influence to acupuncture effect. (Fig.15)

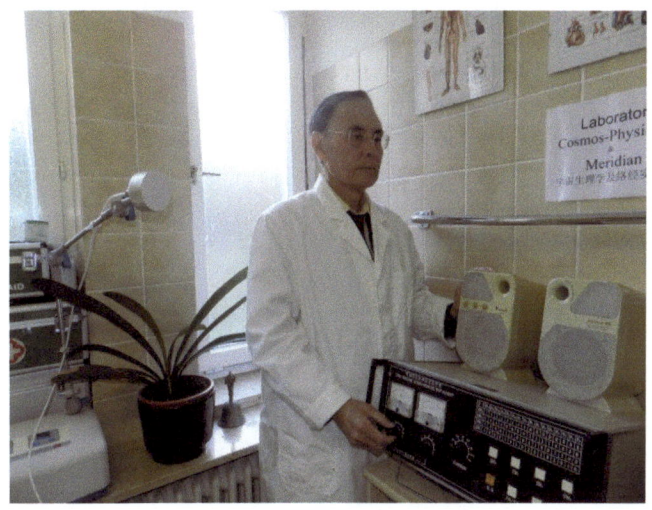

Fig.15 Author is regulating the bionic infrasonic radiator and other spectrum instruments (sonic, micro-wave and infrared, etc.) in Cosmos-Physiology & Meridian Simulative Laboratory

1.6. Bio-Wave and Concept of "Qi" in Traditional Chinese Medicine

In recent half century, much more scientists pay attention to the liquid-crystal structure of macro molecule in membrane of cell (Fig. 16). In 1972 Singer and Nicolson supplied the "Fluid mosaic model", 1975 Wallach put forward the "Crystal lattice mosaic model", 1977 Jain and White advanced the "Plate mosaic model".

31

When the membrane is in the situation of liquid-crystal the small molecules and protein are easy to pass through the membrane; when it is only in crystal situation the small molecules and protein could not go through the membrane.

The bio-wave can make the plate of the liquid-crystal membrane in the vibrational situation, enhance the motion and mobility of membrane's lipid bilayers, and realize the materials and information full exchange and guarantee metabolism of cells.

With high times electron-microscope, the views of wave movement phenomena of membrane in epithelium cells of small intestine could be observed.

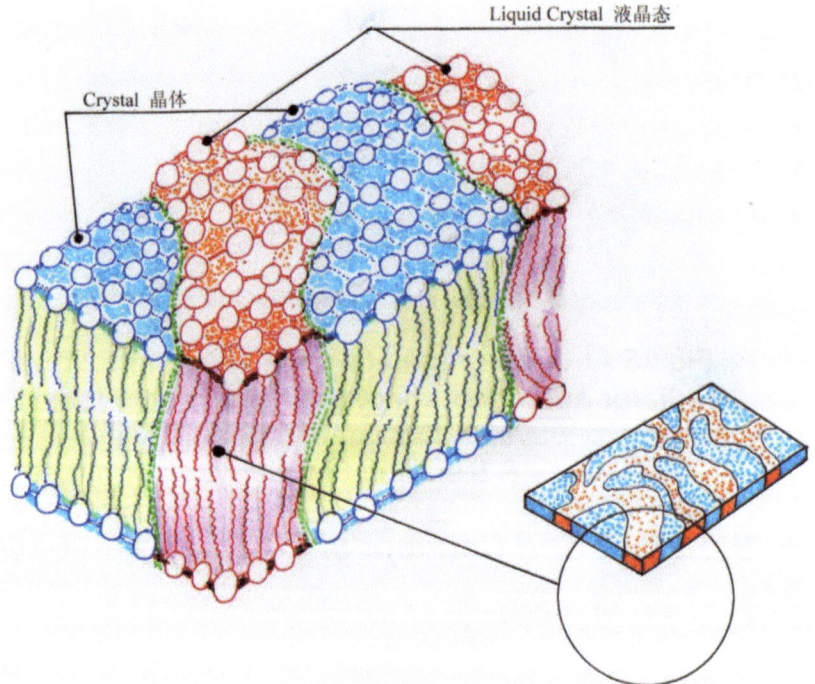

Fig. 16 Tectonics of Liquid Crystal Plate of Cell's Membrane

The "**Dynamics of Wave to Cell**" put forward by author could help to crack the principle of life of cell. The principle of "Dynamics of Wave to Cell" is to research the cellar life phenomena in the

32

background of bio-wave's action to cell, and to research cell's movable situation, but static situation". It may reveal the new principle of physiology and pathology which have not been known until now.

Fig. 19 is the total model of the "Bio- Physics-Mathematics of Bio-Wave" in meridian. According this model, the phase velocity of bio-wave in the human's body can be calculated about 1000 – 1600 m/sec, the amplitude of membrane is about in the scale of nano, the energy is about in the spectrum of erg. Until now the calculation is roughly, because much more parameters of physics and mechanics of human' body have not been researched and measured, which can we estimated only. The author hopes in this field the scientists could research and make more experiments to establish precisely data-base.

Chinese medicine and European medicine developed with different directions: TCM carried on holism, systematology and differentiation with the direction of meridian science, and European medicine promoted reduction science with the base of anatomy. We believe on the **bridge of cell molecular biology** which was arisen before 20 years, combining the theory of bio-wave, a new and more effective and reasonable medicine of prevention and therapy could be established by the scientists, TCM doctors and European doctors. (Fig. 53)

Meridian phenomenon is a "Field Effect of Bio-Wave". To research meridian should be under the thinking of "Field of Life" but "Anatomy Structure". The spreading of vibration and wave in the body is so called "Qi" of TCM before 2000 years, and the "Xu" in TCM is the blood circulation and micro-circulation. These vibration and bio-wave guarantees the substance exchange and metabolism between micro-circulation and cell's membrane, and also guarantees the transmit of signal and transmitter between nerve (including endocrine also) systems and cells of organs.

TCM has paid much more attention to the importance of **"Qi"** and **"Xue"** for 2500 years before. From this point of view, where the Qi and Xue could fully arrived into the tissues or organs, where would no symptoms appear and man will keep healthy. **Qi's running is just the Bio-wave's conduction in meridian.** The unobstructed conduction of bio-wave Qi in the meridian is the guarantee for the running of Xue (blood micro-circulation) into the tissues and organs abundantly. Chinese medicine adopts acupuncture, massage, cupping and moxabition, etc. to cure diseases. Its aim is to enhance and regulate the bio-wave in meridian for the balance of Qi and Xue. The using of Chinese herbs is also to regulate Qi and Xue with the action of bio-chemistry to reach the therapeutic aim.

The production of bio-wave relies on the normal discharge of cardiac electric current and cerebral central nerve current, therefore the health of human body, in the last analysis, depends on the good physiologic situation of heart and brain, a physique heart and an intelligent brain are the bases of healthy of person.

1.7. The action of solar emission to the bio-wave

We have discussed the influence of the field of earth magnet to the bio-wave, indeed the emission of sun also produces propagation of sound wave in the earth (solar wind), and the **Magnet acoustic wave** and **Alfvén wave** can also act on the body (Fig. 17).

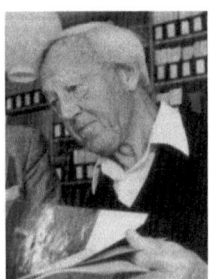

Fig. 17 Hannes Olof Alfvèn, Sweden 1908-1995,1970 Nobel Prize Winner

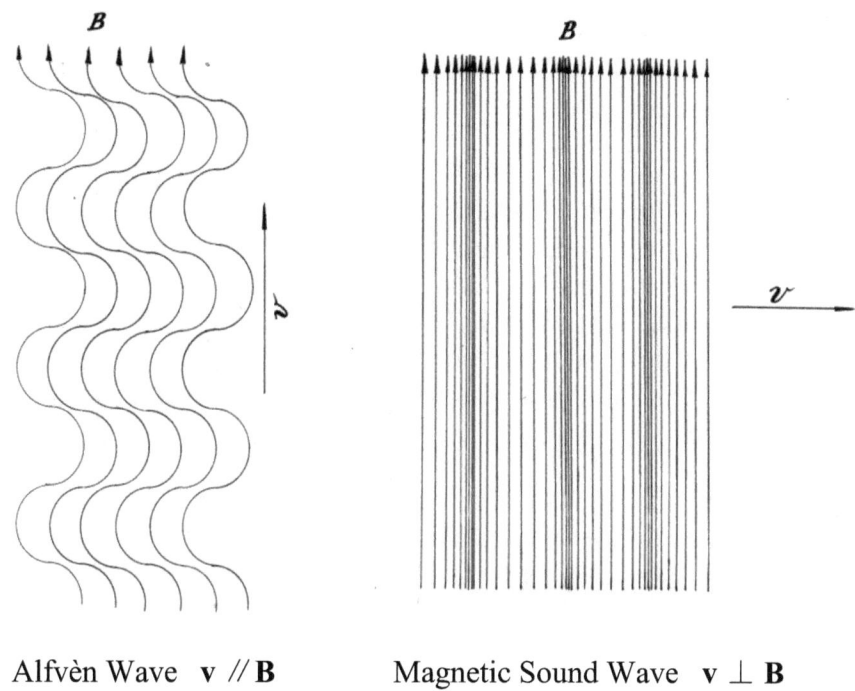

Alfvèn Wave **v // B**   Magnetic Sound Wave **v ⊥ B**

Fig. 18 Alfvèn Wave (transversal wave) and Magnetic Sound Wave (longitudinal wave) which are from the plasma of Solar Wind

In1963 Sweden scientist Alfvèn discovered the Magnetic Sound Wave and Ion Sound Wave which all are produced by the plasma of solar wind, their frequencies are within sound wave spectrum. Alfvèn wave's conductive direction is parallel with magnetic field (transversal wave); Magnetic sound wave's direction is vertical with magnetic field (langitudinal wave). They also have some action for producing bio-wave in the human body. (Fig. 18) The detail describtion will be written in another book.

1.8 The Origin of Earth's Life

Generally speaking the guarantees of the existing of earth's life are: Air, Water and Sunshine. But from my research there is the fourth condition, which is the Geo-Magnet.

Of cause the "magnetic sheath" (Fig. 6) formed by geo-magnetic field is very important, which protects the air and water of earth. Otherwise they could be blown away to cosmos by Solar Wind.

The second reason is the Bio-Wave theory. Prof. David Dunlop (Geo-physist, Toronto University) discovered the oldest geo-magnet greenstone belt in South Africa, which has the age of 3500 million years (<Science> 05, Mar. 2011). Coincidentally the oldest microorganism in old rock also has 3500 million years age, which were discovered in South Africa and Australia. That means the origin of earth's life is accompanied with the produce of geo-magnetic field.

From my research of bio-wave, the production of earth's bio-wave of life is based on the appearance of geo-magnet. **This illustrates that except water, air and sunshine, the geo-magnetic field is the fourth element for life guarantee. This is the most important discovery by author in the research of meridian. I think this discovery is with huge significance in the theory of life science.**

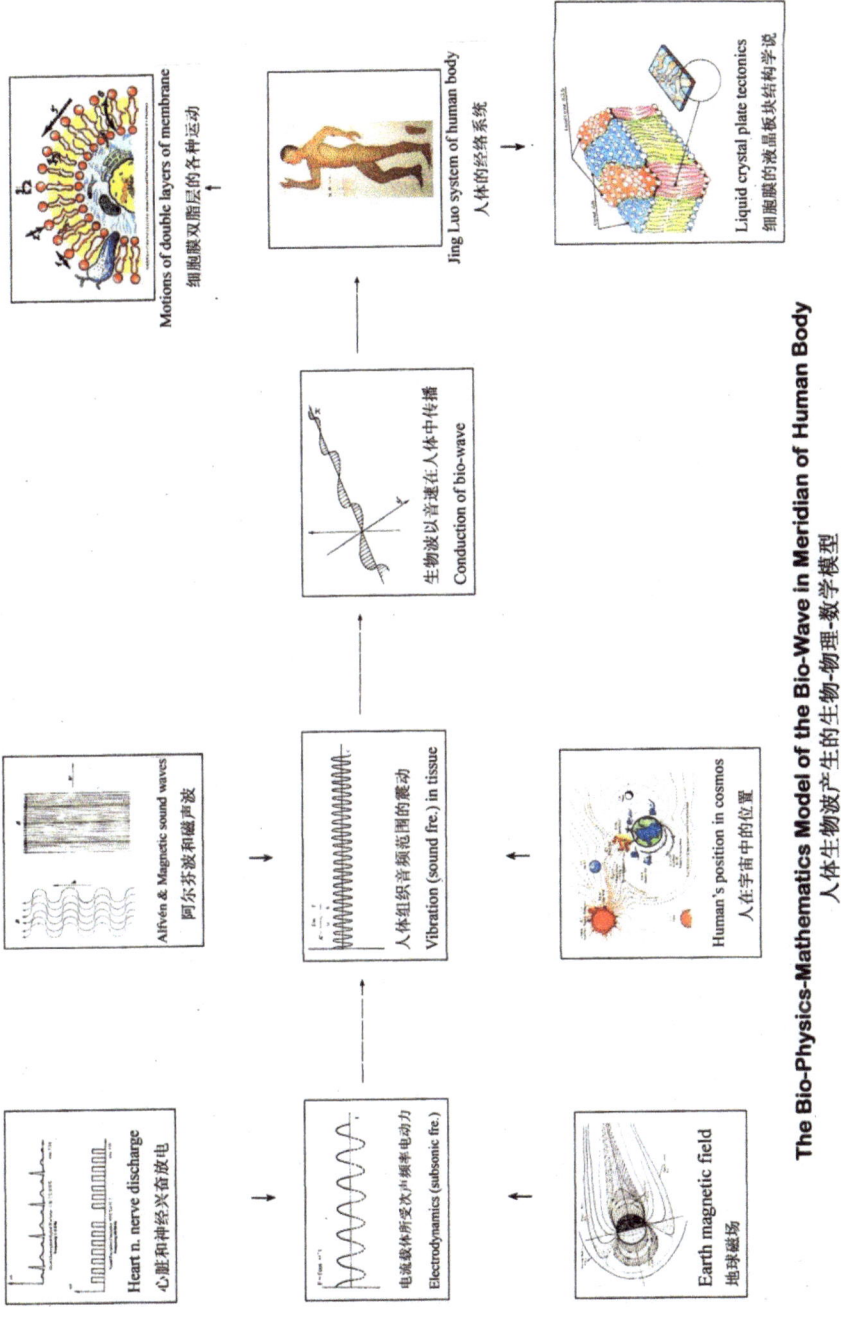

Fig. 19   The Bio-Physics-Mathematics Model of Bio-Wave in Meridian

2. The Theoretical Basis of Cellular Molecular Biology for Acupuncture

2.1. "Standing Wave" Produced by Acupuncture Changes the Physiological Situation of Cell

The Bio-Waves of human body conduct along the meridians, the Acu-points in meridian are the regions with much more energy density of wave. When needles insert into the tissue of Acu-points, the phenomenon of **"Interference Wave"** appears, then the **Standing wave** is produced and makes the vibration's amplitude much bigger, the "nodal point effect" becomes stronger, at same time the standing wave increases the action to the membrane, plasma and nuclear of cell, finally a serious phenomenon of physiology happens.

The follows are the explanation how the standing wave produced. When the needles insert muscle, for example in point A and B (Fig. 20), the conducting bio-wave meets the stainless-steel needle. The reflective coefficient of wave at different mediums (tissue and steel) is very high (about 99%). The amplitude C of reflective wave Y2 is same with the incident wave Y1, the maximum amplitude of the synthetic interference wave Y should be 2C (two times of C) in the wave peak, but in point A and B should be 0. The mathematical derivation is as follows:

Y1 is the amplitude of the incident wave, Y2 is the reflective wave,

$$Y_1 = C \cos 2\pi \left(\frac{t}{T} - \frac{x}{\lambda} \right) \qquad Y_2 = C \cos 2\pi \left(\frac{t}{T} + \frac{x}{\lambda} \right)$$

The amplitude of the synthetic standing wave:

$$Y = Y_1 + Y_2 = 2\ C\ \cos\ \frac{2\ \pi}{\lambda}\ x\ \cos\ \frac{2\ \pi}{T}\ t$$

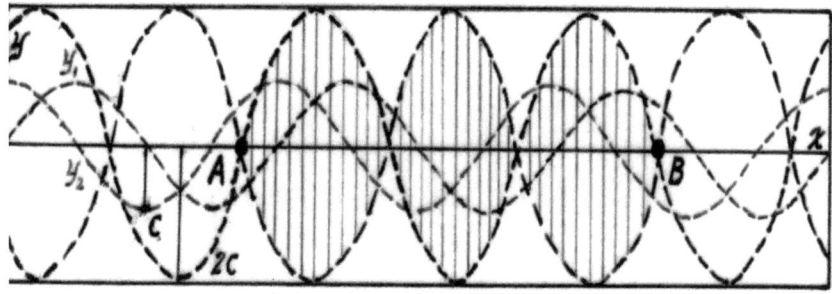

Fig. 20 In Acupuncture the Bio-Wave becomes Standing Wave

At this time the bio-wave doesn't conducts forward, the simple harmonic motion appears at every point between A and B. The maximum amplitude is 2C in the middle point. The Standing Wave is formed and increases the motion and fluidity of cells, changes the metabolic situation of cells.

The stronger vibration of cell makes the human body enters into **"Excited Situation"** or **"Acupuncture Situation"** (see Fig.14). Under the function of stronger acoustic wave, the situation of membrane, F-actin, the microtube in plasma and the nucleus have been changed obviously. The membrane becomes discontinuity and thick, the F-actin and microtubes become longer and thicker, the nucleus becomes circular and bigger. All the exchanges are illustrated the situation of the cells become active. The capability of metabolism of cells is reinforced.

At this time along meridian every point vibrates at original position, the wave conducts no longer along the meridian. This phenomenon induces many important changes of cell's function, such as Synapes block in acupuncture analgesia and anesthesia, etc.

39

Chinese Acupuncture includes needle insertion (Fig.42), laser acupuncture (Fig. 43) and moxibustion (Fig.44, Fig. 45). Through stimulating the Acu-points of meridian by needle or burning moxa stick, the "Qi" and "Xue" (Blood) of body could be regulated and enhanced, the immunity and self reha capability would be strengthened, and the illness will be recovered. Chinese Massage (Fig. 46) and Cupping (Fig. 47) have the same fuction as acupuncture.

2.2. The Changing of Function of Cell by Behaviour of Calsium Ion in Acupuncture

2.2.1. The Important Significance of Discovery of "Enrichment of Ca++", "Vibration of Ca++" and "Wave of Ca++" in Acupuncture

In 1970s Chinese doctors GUO Yi, ZHANG Chun Xi, XU Tang Ping, etc. had found the phenomena of enrichment and oscillation of Ca++ in the acu-points when acupuncture operated. They have researched this phenomenon about more than 10 years.

In the period of 1980 – 1995 bio-physists and molecular biologists J. Sneyd, M. J. Sanderson, J. B. Michael and B. Alberts, etc. found the follows "Calcium Wave" phenomena: as stimulating a cell with mechanic forms, the density of calcium irons increase obviously innerior the cell. At same time the calcium ions appear oscillation. When stimulating one single cell, the neighbor cells also appear the phenomena of vibrating and enriching of calcium ions. This vibration can spread and diffuse continuously to neighbor cells. This is the "Calcium Wave".

They also found a very important phenomena in their experiments that this wave can spread either in the homo-cells or can spread between different kinds of cells, such as from derma to muscle, organ, bone, etc. by the interstitials".

Fig. A is from the thesis: J. Sneyd etc. 《Mechanesmus of Calcium Oscillations and Waves: Quantutative Analysis》. FASEB Journal 1995091463-1472

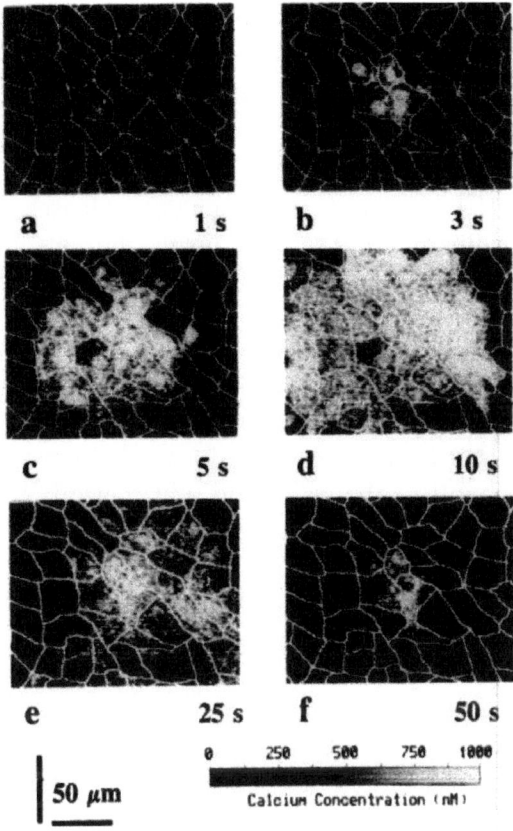

Fig.A. An experiment of calcium wave between cells.

The series images from a – f show the changing of calcium ions of epithelium cells within the space and different times. This changing is beginning from one cell which was stimulated by mechanisms in a pacing point. The white point is the position stimulated. The white lines are the boundaries of cells. (Fig.A,a) After stimulation the wave of calcium ions spread to total culture dish towards every direction. After 10 sec. the wave spreads 60% area of the total cells. In every boundary of cells, the waves stay about 0.5 – 1 second.

Once the wave over, the density of calcium ions decreases quickly. The part of white color is the area of enrichment of calcium ions.

After a big amount of experiments and computer simulations, the result of analysis of this thesis are:

1. The wave has no relation with the osmotic coefficient of calcium ions between cells. Generally speaking calcium ions do not spread between cells.

2. IP3 (inositol triphosphate) releases calcium ions (from cellular organs) only inside the cell and not spread outside the membrane.

3. The Calcium Wave has no relation with IP3 and calcium ions.

At least the author in this thesis put forward a question, "We don't realize what control the velocity and period of the wave's alignment?"

The author realize that the dynamics of calcium wave is not from calcium ion and IP3. The mechanical stimulation makes the calcium ions releasing (MOCs) from the calcium stores (inclusive microtube, F-Actin in the cell and interstitial outside the cell) and enriching in the cell. At same time the bio-wave (specially the Standing Wave which is also induced by the action of the mechanisms) induces calcium ions' oscillation and the spreading in the calcium waves. This is because the starting of bio-wave is also from the mechanical stimulation at same time. We should explain the production of calcium wave with the theory of **bio-physics but bio-chemistry**. It is the bio-wave which induces the appearing of enrichment and vibration of IP3 and calcium ions and the enrichment of calcium irons between neighbor cells one by one.

In 1987 Lansman etc. found when epithelium cell is stimulated by mechanical drawing, the calcium tunnels open, i.e. "Calcium ions' tunnels of Mechanical activation MOCs". (The other tunnels are ROCs, SMOCs, and VOCs etc.)

The density of calcium ion in the interstitial is over 1000 times than inside the cell. The permeability ratio of Ca^{++} to Na^+ is about 6 : 1. When cell is drawn by mechanical stimulation (such as needle, knife, acupuncture, etc.) the tunnels MOCs are opened and a big amount of calcium ions pour into cells' plasma from interstitial through membrane, and then enrichment and oscillation of ions are occurring by the strong action of bio-wave (Standing Wave). Due to the difference of density of ions between cells is very low, it is not possible that the calcium ions could diffuse between neighbor cells. This is the reason that J. Sneyd did not find moving of calcium ions between cells.

We must emphasize "Calcium Wave" and "Bio-Wave" are two different concepts completely. Bio-Wave (Standing Wave) is produced by the interaction between the geo-magnetic field and the electric current of heart and brain. Calcium Wave is produced by the opening of MOCs and dynamics of bio-wave. But the two phenomena could be traced to the same origin, i.e. the mechanical stimulation. In Chinese medicine, the stimulation has many forms, such as Acupuncture, massage, cupping, etc.

Above is the Vitro-situation of enrichment and oscillassion of calcium iron. About Vivo experiments, in 1970s Chinese scientists and doctors has found the phenomena of centripetal and vibration of calcium ions at points along the meridian when acupuncture operated. 2010s scientists of Hong Kong Uni. found the transversal acoustic wave and enriched calcium irons along the meridian with NMR experiment when acupuncture needles thrust into the body. These foundations have very important scientific significance for basic theory of acupuncture with Cellular molecular biology.

2.2.2. The Special Physiological Function of Calcium Ion

In 1883 Dr. Ringer found when persusion of Calcium oxide into the non-pulsing heart, the heart could be recovered pulse. He also found Ca^{++} could enhance the contractility and prolong the time of systole of heart. After then scientists began to research the important fuction of Calcium ions.

Round the nucleus of atom Ca20 has 4 orbits of electron, i.e. 2-8-8-2. There are full electrons in the second and third orbits. Two electrons are in the fourth orbit. Calcium is a metal with 2-valence electron. Comparing with other ions, Calcium ion has bigger ion radium, higher negative electric charge and more electric charge density. The electric-chemistry gradient of Ca^{++} in the double side of membrane is higher than other ions. For example, the density of Ca^{++} outside the membrane of myocardial fibers is about 10-3 g per liter. But interior membrane is 10-7 g per liter. This means the difference is 10000 times.

When membrane is stimulated by machinery or electric, under the action of depolarization, the tunnels of membrane open and the calcium stores release Ca^{++}. The density of Ca^{++} interior of membrane increase instantaneously, and many important physiological phenomena happen. With same conditions, due to Ca^{++} is 2-valences positive ion, the moving velocity of Ca^{++} is 2 times as other one valence ions, such as K^{+}, Na^{+}. Interior of membrane the dissociation and combination of Ca^{++} with other molecules are very quickly., Ca^{++} can pass through membrane very easily which has very important significance in metabolic of cell and in the transmission of nerve signal.

Calcium ion can induce important physiological activities, some times by calcium ions themselves; much more times by protein combined Calcium or accepters of calcium. Calmodulin (CaM) is the most important Calbindin Protein which has very high avidity with calcium. It is a sensor of calcium interior cell and arranges very widely. CaM is a oligopeptide composed by 148 amino acid residue (from Cheung) and molecular weight is 16700 Dalton. There are more than 10 kinds of enzymes are affinity with calcium. The physiological function of CaM is very important and widely.

The physiological function are as follows:

1. Regulate the activity of myodial cell. The heart electro-excitation by depolarization and contract couple. This is owing to calcium ion releasing from SR sarcoplasma reticulum.

2.   The excitive and contractive couple of muscle activity is induced by calcium ion which regulates the interaction of actin and myosin.

3.   The up-afferent signal of sense organ and pain, as well as the down-afference of nerve instruction all have relation with calcium ion in synapes. The physiological process of synapse has relation with calcium ions for transmitters releasing.

4.   The follows physiological activities all have relation with the calcium ions:

fluidity of plasma, regulation of cellular skeleton, mobility and ablation of micro-fiber and tube, pilus' moving, mobility and dissolution of cytocyst, releasing of transmitters, etc.

5.   Retention of fluidity and mobility of liquid-crystal membrane, guarantee of electro-potential of cells, as well as protection of the passing through membrane of multi- kinds of ions.

6.   Increasing the activity of enzymes.

7.   Secreting of hormone.

8.   Guarantee the synthesis, storage, replication, transcription of genetic materials, cell's division and hyperplasia.

9.   Fertilization of ovum.

10.   etc.

Therefore, calcium ions' enrichment and oscillation in acupuncture make the function of cells changing with a big scale, then realize the therapy for many kinds of illness.

Of cause calcium ion also has negative influences. Such as the exceed quantity of calcium ions in cardiac cell will induce anoxemia of myocardium, as traumatic cerebral oedema the exceed calcium ions will make accelerative death of nerve cells, etc.

From the point of TCM calcium ion is belong to "Yang" (energy), when the action of calcium ion is exceeded strong, the balance of "Ying" (organs) and "Yang" will be broken, the "excess of Yang" happens and relative diseases will appear.

Acupuncture not only produce the enrichment and oscillation for calcium ions, but also induce the characters changing of other ions (for example H^+, Na^+, K^+, Mg^{++}, etc.), proteins and macro molecules. Author realize those phenomena should be researched deeply also.

Just as the speech by Dr. Hammerschlag (biological chemist of origin medical institute, Oregon University), "acupuncture is a challenging to the model of modern biology, the effect of acupuncture should have relation with bio-medicine. In addition, it is not easy to explain some phenomena of acupuncture with mechanisms of neurography realized now. So the transmission of signal of acupuncture may be conducted through part of physiology and self-regulation, but nerve system". Author agree above opinion, meridian and nerve are two different systems absolutely.

2.2.3. The Explain for two Opposite Diseases can be therapied by same Acu-Point in Acupuncture

The Magical effect of acupuncture is two completely different symptoms or diseases could be therapied with same acu-points. For example, when needles insert the two points of Nei Guan (PC 6 内关) and Qu Chi (LI 11 曲池) (Fig.21) either bradycardia or tachycardia all can be cured; either hypertension or hepotension also all can be cured. The wonder is decided by the theory of bio-wave and the special characters of cell's membrane. When patient enters into "acupuncture excited situation", the movement and fluidity of membrane are increased,

K$^+$ flows out of membrane more in acupuncture, the electro-potential is higher, the exchange of substances, energy and information are enhanced. At same time the calcium ions are released from Ca^{++} stores much more, Ca^{++} make the activity of cardiac muscle stronger, thus the tachycardia and hypotension could be cured.

Relatively for bradycardia, due to the stronger bio-wave by acupuncture induces the hyperpolarization of membrane and increases threshold value of depolarization, the membrane could not be discharged, and the bradycardia could be cured. On the other hand, for hypertension patient due to the action of bio-wave, the membrane of smooth muscle of coronary artery and arteria vessel of all the body increase mobility and fluidity, the elasticity of vascular wall is increased, thus, the blood pressure will be reduced.

From above illustration, we could know the human body has the capability of self-regulation and self-weighting in the therapy by acupuncture.

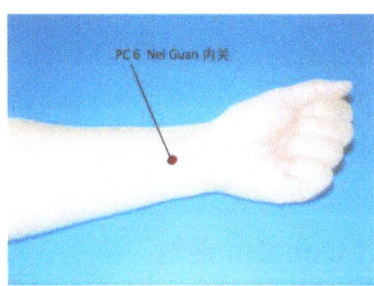 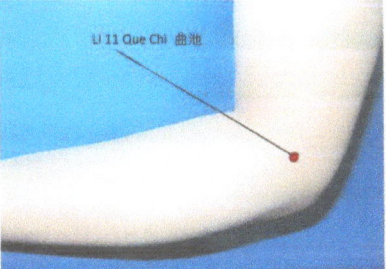

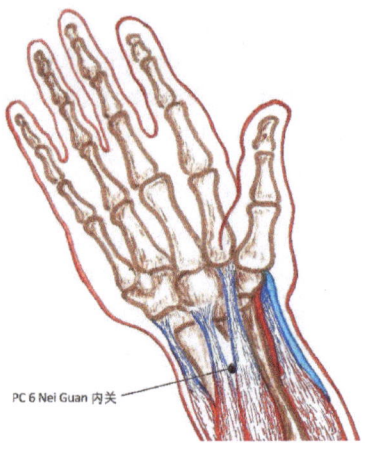

PC 6 Nei Guan 内关

Fig.21a Acu-Point PC 6 Nei Guan 内关

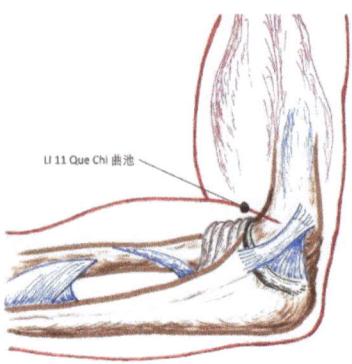

LI 11 Que Chi 曲池

Fig.21b. Acu-Point LI 11 Que Chi 曲池

3. The Principle of Cellular Molecular Biology for Acupuncture Analgesia and Anesthesia

In 1970 Chinese doctors developed and used acupuncture for anesthesia in operation. To select right meridian and acu-points, the needles are inserted and stimulate the tissue with special strong manual, making the patient has fillings of "acetose, tingling, heavy and distending", the operation can be started, and without narcotic.

In this book author pick forward a new theory of anesthesia which is based on the theory of bio-wave and the interdisciplinary with cellular molecular biology.

3.1 The Production and Transmission for sense of Pain

General speaking the pain transmission has two forms: chemic signal and electric signal, and much more by bio-chemistry. In bio-chemical way the function of nerve transmitter is very important. The transmitter is composed in neuron and stored in nerve end. After depolarization of pre-synapse (due to mechanisms or traumatic stimulation, etc.) calcium ions are released from calcium storages (in intertitial and in micro fible and tube of cell) into cell's plasma. Owing to the function of calcium ion (regulator) the cytocyst moves forward to presynapse membrane, and then fuses with membrane, the exocytosis appears, dozens of kinds of algesthesia transmittels release into the synapse cleft. Then the accepter of post-synapse is excited and the depolarization happens, the signal of pain is conducted into center nerve. From above illustration we could see the importance of calcium ion.

The pain transmission is a much competed process. After nocuous stimulation for example, needle insertion, collision, operation, etc., the sensors (such as of non-myelin sheath C nerve and of A nerve with myelin sheath) excited. When the frequency of stimulation reaches a defined value, the pain will happen. The nocuous stimulation induces depolarization of membrane of nerve ending, the sensor and nocuous cell release bio-chemical substance of pain, which include: 1) ATP, Ach, K^+, etc. from damaged cells; 2) P Substance etc. from sensors; 3) enzyme and synthetic substance from damaged cells and 4) some substance from moving blood. These substances all can induce transmission of the sense of pain. P-substance and Glu. (Glutamic), etc. are contained in C nerve; Glu. Atc. Are contained in A nerve.

Between nucoous sensor of ending and dorsal horn, the transactive function of synapse is very important. The pain-transmission of synapse pass through Aβ, Aδ and C nerve, and reach dorsal horn of spinal cord. P Substance and Glu glutamic acid etc. are contained in C nerve, Glu etc. iare contained in A nerve. These substances are stored in cytocyst of pre-synapse.

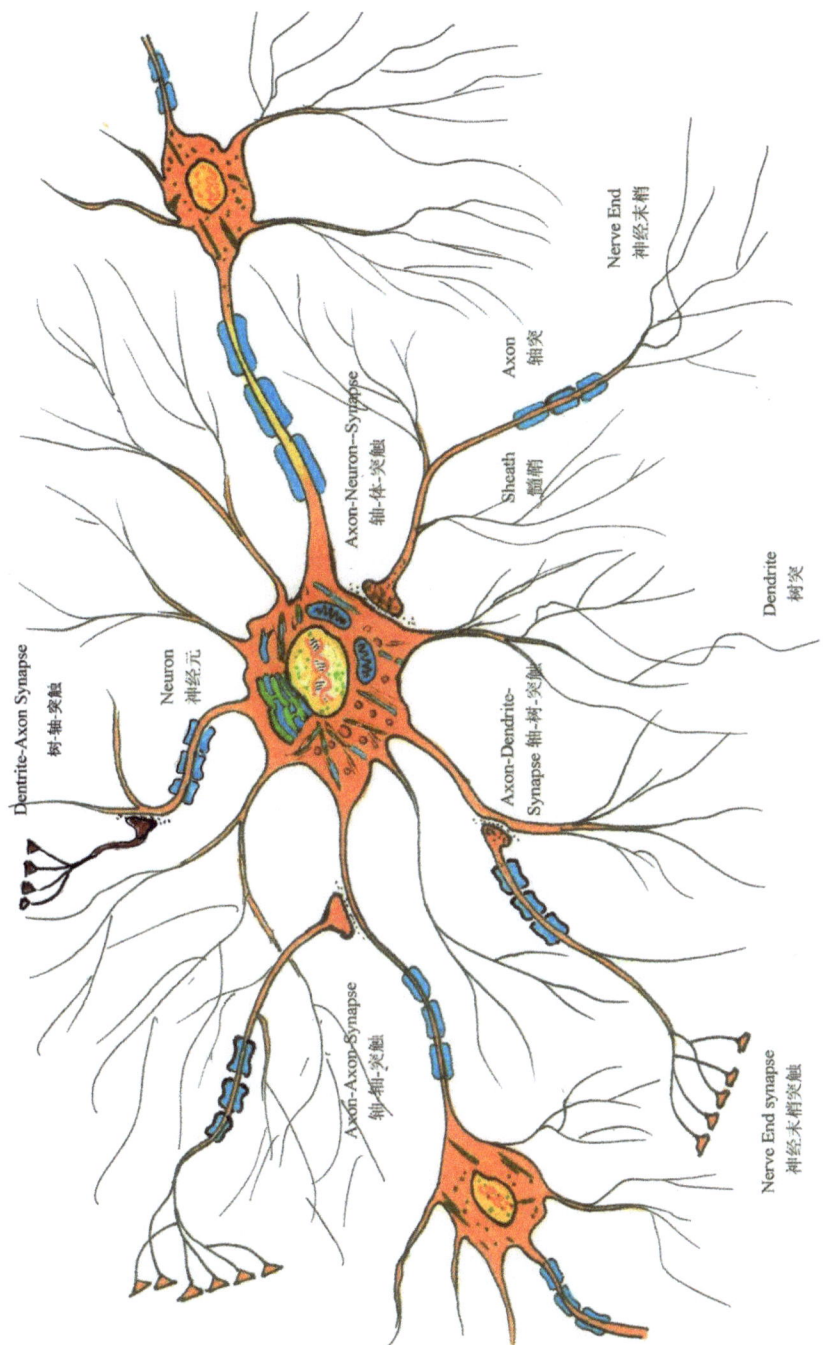

Fig. 22. Function of nerve transmission for Synapse

51

Under the action of Ca^{++} the cytocysts appear the phenomena of exosytosis, these substances are released. These transmitters make membrane of post- synapse opened and depolarization of membrane. This process realizes pain signal reaching the center of nerve. Fig. 22.

The follows are the process of exosytosis phemomena and conduction for sense of pain to the center nerve in detail:

α) Depolarization of nerve end after nocuous stimulated,

β) Outside of membrane of pre-synapse, big amount of Ca^{++} pure into cell through MOCs, VOCs. At same time IP3 also makes cell organ releasing Ca^{++} into plasma. Ca^{++} is 2 valence metal, and have more bio-activity to realize and combine with target enzyme.

γ) Ca^{++} combine with accepter, CaM etc., activate protein kinase relying on Ca^{++}/CaM,

remove and ablate the restriction of cytocyst from skeleton (such as micro-fiber, tube, etc.), the cytocyst is untied from skeleton and drift into the plasma of pre-synapes.

Δ) By the action of Ca^{++}, cytocysts swim to the pre-membrane, the membranes of cytocys and pre-synapes are close to each other. (please see "Machinery regulating vesiele traffic, a major transport system in our cells". James E. Rothman, Randy W. Schekman, Tomas C. Südhof, 2013 Nobel Physiology Preis owners.

ε) The membrane of cytocyst is ablated, exocytosis appears, the pain medium (such as P-substance, ATP, Ach, K^+, etc. more than 50 kinds) well into synapse cleft, these medium fuse with the accepters of post-synapes.

ζ) After the interaction of accepter and ligand in membrane of post-synapse, the tunnels of ions open. (Sometimes ion tunnel formed by accepters directly).

η) The fast-discharge EPSP of post-synapes produces after excited depolarization.

Θ) The pain signal transmitted to the dorsal root of spinal cord and thalamus which is the most important algesia centre.

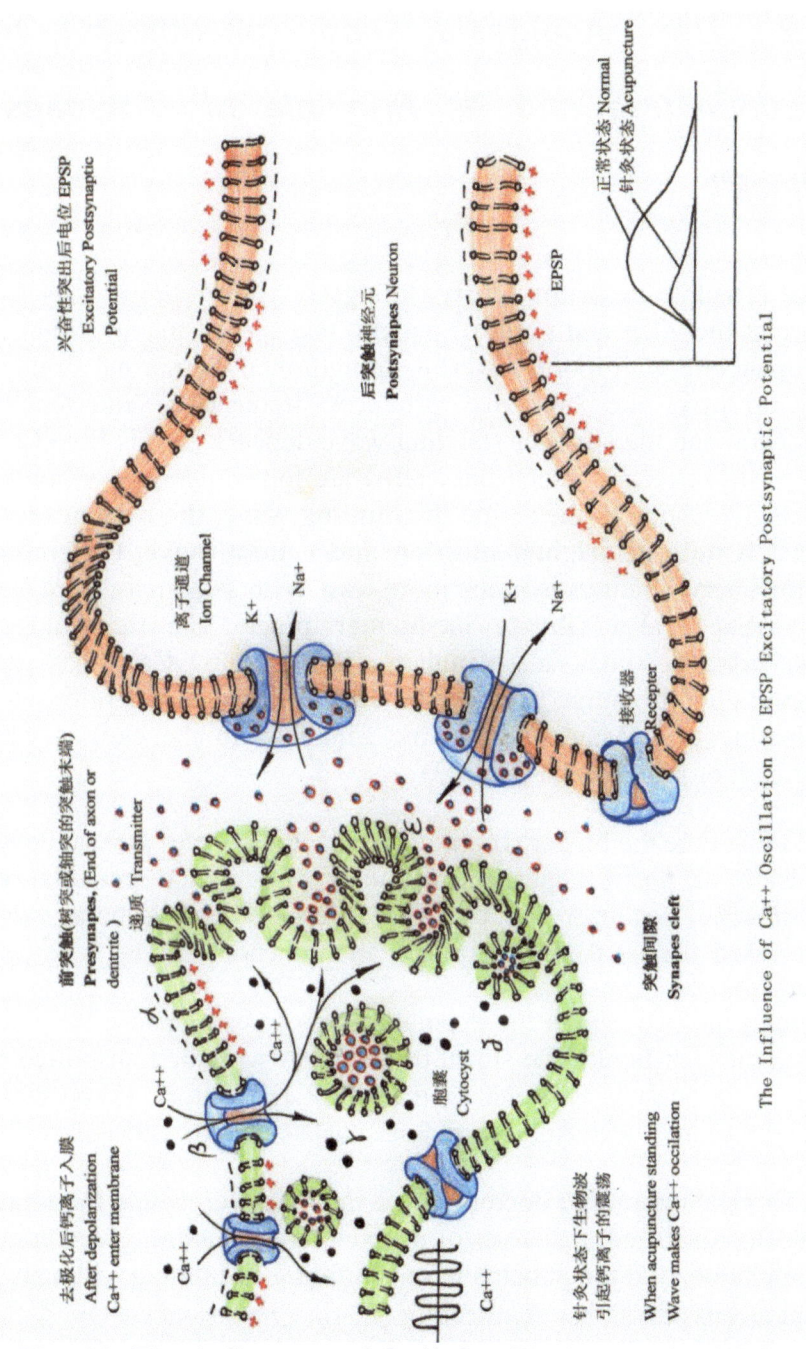

Fig. 23. The Influence of Ca^{++} Oscillation to the EPSP (Excitatory Postsynaptic Potential)

53

3.2 The Analgesia and anesthesia by Acupuncture and its Principle of "Synapse Block"

The principle of **acupuncture Analgesia** is as follows: to select correct meridian and point of patient, use special manipulation of acupuncture with more powerful strength then the normal strength in **therapy**, the bio-wave produces tremendous interference function and the stronger standing wave appears. In this time Ca^{++} in pre-synapse and interstitial nearby are forced damping vibration strongly. Owing to the action of **standing wave, the oscillation of Ca^{++} is only in original position and cannot move**, Ca^{++} reflux into C nerve endings is much more less. With same reason Ca^{++} in pre-synapes also **vibrate in former place**. The threshold of discharge becomes also higher. This means Ca^{++} has not opportunity to move and combine with cytocyst, therefore the releasing of P Material, glutamic acid, etc. to the cleft is very difficult or impossible. (Fig. 23)

At same time the bigger amplitude of Standing waves makes the K^+ outside of post-synapes much more. The resting potential of membrane becomes higher. The threshold of discharge also increased. This is the "Hyperpolarization Phenomena".

Due to the two causes the depolarizition of post-cynapse becomes even more difficult. The signal of pain nearly not be transmitted to the center nerve. This makes the EPSP (Excitatory Postsynapse Potential) into IPSP (Inhibitory Postsynapse Potential) (Fig.25)

In surgical operation, doctors select right acu-points and meridian, use fine qualified mancuver of acupuncture with stronger strength stimulation, and the patients have the filling of tingling and heavy, that means patient has "Collecting Qi" (in China say "De Qi" 得气). In this time the patient is in the "High Energy State" or "Acupuncture Exciting State", only in this time the narcotic drug of surgery is not necessary and the anesthesia of acupuncture is successful.

We must illustrate that if the patient's filling of tingling and heavy disappeared and the Qi deprived, the anesthesia of acupuncture has lost efficiency. This is meaning the situation of patient returns back to the "Normal State" or "Non-Exciting State" and the algesthesia produces again in operation.

In fig. 24 the real line means the pain broken by oscillation of Ca^{++} in original position. The dotted line means pain transmitted by Ca^{++} promoting cytocest moving and fusion with membrane of pre-cynapes, and release much more transmitters into the cleft of synapse.

This is The Anesthesia and Analgesia by Acupuncture and the Principle of Nerve Cellular Molecular Biology (Effect of SYNAPSE BLOCK put forward by author).

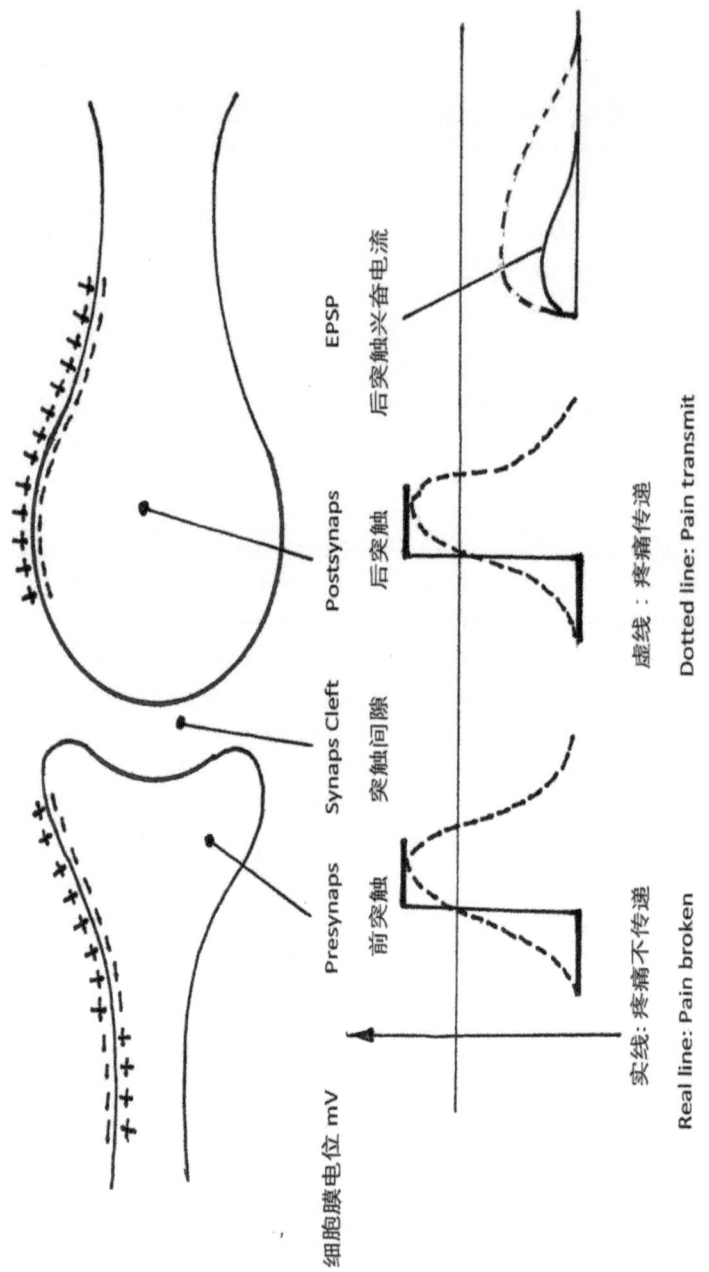

Fig. 24 Owing to Synapse Block, Signal of Pain is cut off to Center Nerve

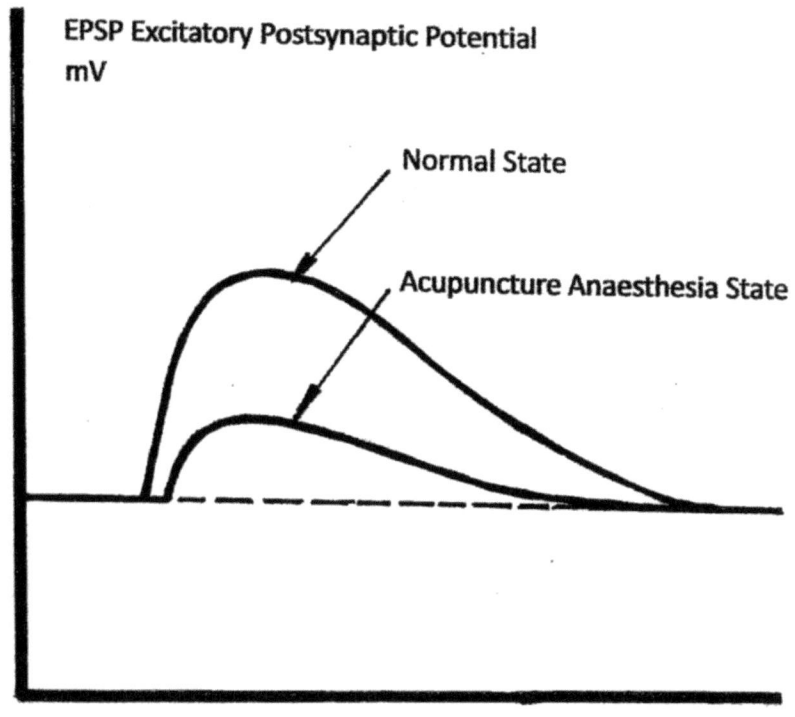

Fig. 25 Excitatory Postsynaptic Potential becomes Inhibitory Postsynapse Potential after Acupuncture Anesthesia

3.3. Opium can be replaced by Acupuncture

This phenomenon is very similar with analgesia of opium. Only to 1973 scientists had known the principle of nerve mechanism of analgesia by opium for analgesia. They discovered opium could increase the K^+ conductivity, make the membrane potential higher, increase the threshold potential, and decrease the ascending current of nerves to center nerve. At same time opium can inhibit Ca^{++} enters in nerve endings, make the fusion of cytosest and membrane impossible, resists the discharge of P Materials and glutamic acid

57

in cleft, EPSP becomes into IPSP (Fig. 25), and realizes the function of analgesia.

3.4. The Summarization of Chapter 2 and Chapter 3

Until now we have discussed the basic principle of acupuncture for therapy, analgesia and anesthesia with the cellular molecular biology.

The following figure is the summarization of the following concepts and basic theory of "Bio-Wave", "Standing Wave", "Therapy Illness by Acupuncture" and "Analgesia and Anesthesia by Acupuncture". The main points are Bio-Wave changes the <u>cellular Situation</u> and Calcium ions change <u>cellular Function.</u> (Fig. 26)

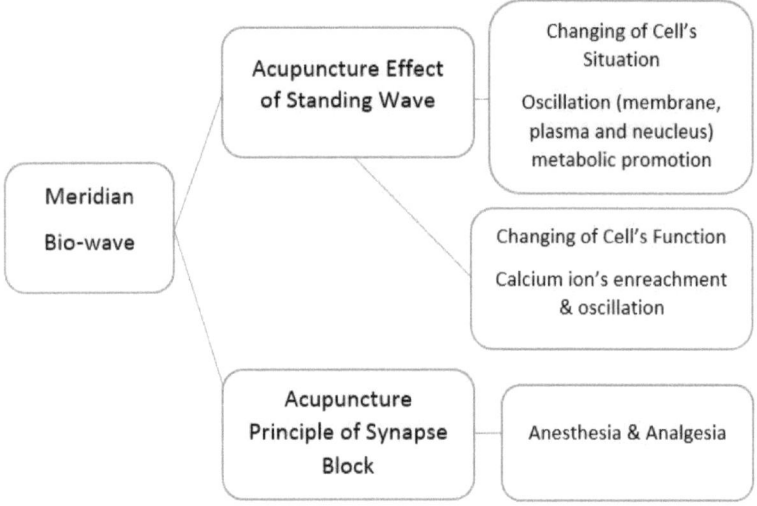

Fig. 26 Summarization: The principle of Cellular Molecular Biology for the Therapy and Analgesia of Acupuncture

4. The Therapy of Qigong for Cancer

4.1. Qigong

Qigong is one of the traditional Chinese methods of cure and rehabilitation for mankind which is belonging of one important part of TCM. With breathing, moving, voicing, thinking and ideal qigong can regulate the bio-wave to strengthen the energy of the body and regulates the meridian of body integrately. The people could reach the situation of total relax and balance, increase the self-immunity and reha capability, and then could cure illness and recover healthy.

Chinese Qigong has had many schools, such as Daoism Qigong, Buddhism Qigong, Confucius Qigong, etc., but which all are based on Daoism Qigong. "Heaven and human are unification" (天人和一) is the principle of Daoism. The people are harmony and united with nature, only when the activities and life of human are coordinated with nature, people could keep health. The Daoism Qigong has continued several thousand years and has had extremely activity, until now it has been contributed to the healthy and rehabilitation for the human.

4.2. The Principle of Cell-Molecular Biology for Curing Cancer by Qigong

Qigong has the special function for anti-cancer. The cancer cell has two characters, one is low electric potential voltage of membrane; another one is anoxybiontic.

Two characters of cancer cells are as follows:

A. Low Electric Potential Voltage of Membrane

It is confirmed that the membrane exists with the situation of liquid crystal organization by the modern cell-molecular biology. With the change of temperature, the membrane transforms between two emphasizes of liquid and crystal. The membrane is composed by double layers lipid molecule, in which cholesterin and glycolipid molecules are very important to guarantee the normal situation of cells, their quantities should be moderate. In higher temperature cholesterin can inhibit fluidity of the membrane; in lower temperature it can increase the fluidity. When the amount of cholesterin and glycolipid molecules decrease and the chain length of glycolipid is too short, the cells will lose the capability of controlling membrane, and the character of flowing of membrane will be aggravated.

When the controlling of membrane fluidity looses, the bio-physics character of cells will be changed. As well-known due to the Na-pump (Na-Ka-ATP pump) and the ion-transmembrane, the normal cells have a transmembrane potential, generally speaking the potential is about -90 mV. It is very important to guarantee the electrolyte balance, metabolism and to maintain of people's life. If the fluidity of membrane increases intensively, the bio-physics effect of ion transmembrane will be broken, the transmembrane potential (absolute value) would be decreased, for example is about -40-50 mV. The decreasing of potential influences the situation of bio-wave directly, which amplitude and energy would become smaller. This could influence the exchange of energy, substance and information between cell interior and outside. At same time the function of cell identification, adhesiveness, growing and differentiation will be cut down, then a big amount of immature cells are divided and produced, the canceration of cells will happen.

B. Anoxybiontic

One of various character of metabolism of cancer cells is reduction of breathing capability and increasing of glycolysis. The quantity of mitochondrion in cancer cell is less than normal cell. The enzyme system of electron transforms chain and the content of ATP are reduced. As well-known mitochondrion is the important place of energy transfer and supplying energy for cells. If the supply of ATP only by anaerobic glycolysis, one glucose molecule can supply two

ATP only, but by mitochondrion, one glucose molecule can supply 36 pieces of ATP.

In the modern research of reversion and division of cancer cell, it has been shown that the cancer cells are produced due to the normal cells' phenotype are impeded in its special maturity period. For example, of acute fine grain leukemia，owing to the bad living environment of cells (radiation, toxicosis, oxygen deficit, mental depression, etc.), big number of immature leukocytes are differentiated desperately. Therefore, we should not say, "Cancer cells are anoxybionic cells", we should say, "Cancer cells are deformity differentiation in the anoxia environment". And we should not say, "Cancer illness is the first murderer of human", should say, "Cancer is the production that human could not deal discreetly with self-body, organs and cells".

4.3. The Therapy of cancer by Guo Lin Qigong

Qigong, especially the Guo Lin Qigong which was created by famous Qigong grand master Ms. Guo, Lin (1910-1984) of China in 1970, has its distinctive function to against these two problems to cure cancer. In the extremely difficult 1970 period of China (Cultural Revolution), grand Qigong master Guo Lin began to teach the Qigong therapy for the patients of cancer (Fig.27).

《 Huang Di Nei Jing 黄帝内经》 appointed, "grand illness need great catharsis". Cancer is crisis and big illness, even if the patients are very weak, Guo Lin recognized that at first the catharsis method must be adopted. On the basis of Daoism Qigong principle and her own experience, Ms. Guo Lin created a new method of breath of "Wind Breathing". The patients use nasal cavity to breath with the rhythmus of "Breathe in — Breathe in — Breathe out". Even if the patients were very weak she still let them to enlarge the action of breath. Big amount of oxygen could be inhaled into the patients which can restrain the growing of cancer cells and at same time make the cancer cells transform to normal cells.

At same time due to the electro-physiological activity of respiration center nerve systems are enhanced, the action of bio-wave will be strengthened and the environment of cells is improved.

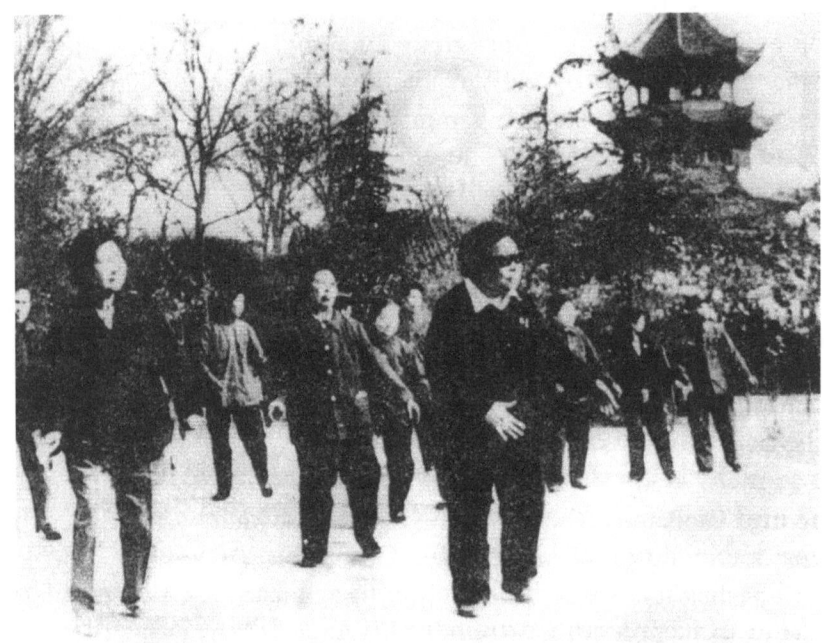

Fig. 27 In 1970 Great Master Ms. Guo Lin taught the patients Qigong

On the other hand, the different regularity moves of hand, feet, head and trunk produce bio-electric currents of body, which currents are induced by the interaction between the Geo-Magnet field and the movement of patient. These currents stimulate and increase the resting potential of membrane, and make the metabolism stronger between membrane and micro-circulation. The glycolysis is restrained, the energy exchange of mitochondrion is enhanced, ATP is produced enough, and the cells transform to cancer cells will be prevented.

Generally, Qigong could be divided two kinds: **"Dong Gong"** (动功 Action Pattern Exercise) and **"Jing Gong"** (静功 Silence Pattern Exercise). The patients with not critical illness can exercise Action Pattern. But the cancer patients, specially the serious cancer patients are very weak; they could not exercise with Action Pattern of Qigong. The Silence Pattern Qigong is mainly with methods of sensing and thinking, it is difficult for the patients of beginning to learn. So Master Guo Lin created **"Zou Gong"** (走功 Walking Pattern Exercise) for cancer patients. The Walking Pattern is situated between Action and silence Pattern. The **Wind Breathing** is accompanied with the exercise of walking of two legs, to finish the 4 steps （**Xi, Xi, Hu, Zhuan 吸吸呼转**）continuous moves of **"Breathe in with nose"** — **"Breathe in with nose"** — **"Breathe out with mouth"** — **"Turn of Head and Trunk"**. When patient exercises "Breathe in", the tip of toe should stick up, that could regulate the Kidney Meridian. When exercises "Turn of Head and Truck" the head and back should be turned to out side direction, which could regulate the Meridian of liver and spleen. With this "Walking Pattern Exercise" the patients can breathe much more oxygen, at same time, the harmony moves of hand, feet, trunk, legs and tip toe can regulate the 12 meridians making bio-wave, Qi and Blood conductivity, promote metabolism, increase self immunity function, and then to eliminate and remove the evil of cancer.

Except "Zou Gong", Master Guo Lin also paid much more attention to the "Sound Gong". According the "Five Element" Principle (see 0.2.2) Five Sound Tone (Gong 宫, Shang 商, Jiao 角，Zhi 徵 and Yü 羽) corresponds to Five Organs (Wu Zang: Spleen, Lungs, Liver, Heart and Kidney). The patient vocalizes with one of the five tones to stimulate the correspond organ which could be induced resonance. The bio-wave with the meridian of this organ would enhance the action to the cells of this organ to reach the effect of therapy.

According the illness situation patients can exercise 10 minutes of this Walking Exercise of Guo Lin Qigong at beginning, after a rest, walking again to 20 minutes or half hour. To exercise every day will get good curing effect. Guo Lin Qigong is different with other

Qigong, it advocates the principle of differentiation of TCM. It adopts different forms of breath and actions for different patients, different illness situation and different illness period. Even if for one patient, different form are adopted in different periods of therapy. For example, Guo Lin Qigong uses different programs to different cancer patient and to different courses of treatment. So, the better and quicker effect of therapy could be reached.

Guo Lin Qigong has been used widely not only in China, but also spread all over the world. In Europe there are much more Qigong masters to teach Guo Lin Qigong and per thousands of patients of cancer have been profited by Guo Lin Qigong. In the recent ten years, Köln Guo Lin Qigong Akademie has trained dozens Guo Lin Qigong masters who are the key members to teach this Qigong in Europe (Fig. 28. Website: guolin-neuqigong.de).

The following cases are two cancer patients have recovered healthy by exercising Guo Lin Qigong in Germany, one is a patient with mammary cancer and metastatic lunge cancer, lympha cancer, vertebra cancer; another is a patient with chronic leukemia. The follows are the accounts of patients' own words.

Case 1

Name: Ms. M. Maldener, born in 1958. Saarbrücken, RP, Germany

Diagnose: Mammary cancer, and metastatic lunge, lympha and vertebra cancers.

In 2005 when I was 47 years old, the mammary cancer has been tested up in my body. Due to the illness time is too long, the cancers have been appeared in metastatic lunge, lympha and vertebra. There are three tumours in lungs, one is big and two are smaller. At that time, I had serious pain whole the body, nearly had not any capability of movement. The result of diagnose was very bad, Doctors said I only could live to the end of the year and suggested me at first accepted chemotherapy before operation. From May to November 2005 there are multi-times therapies of chemo and antibiotic. In this period one of my relatives told me a health Qigong. I tried to do 40 minutes exercise of this Qi Gong every day. I felt some benefit to lysis the side function of chemotherapy.

After then I found the "Guo Lin Qigong" in internet, this Qigong has special effect for cancers. In 2006 after the operation of mammary cancer, I took part in course of Guo Lin Qigong in Landau by Frau Li Wang. I had studied different exercises of Guo Lin Qigong: "Natural Go", "Middle and fast Go", "Special fast Go", "One step, Two steps and Three steps" (Fig.29). After the course finished, every day morning I exercised the above moves outside and in afternoon I exercised "Fixed step", "Ascending, descending, opening and closing" and "Silence Gong". I insisted to exercise Guo Lin Qigong, and benefited much. Until now I still live in the world! Now the suffering of pain has been alleviated more, and can do some works. The two small tumours have been disappeared to a miracle, and the big one also has become smaller.

Owing to the effect is so good, I always think and observe the effective results in other fields for Guo Lin Qigong. Really, I found my lympha system has been better. My 12 lympha nodes used to be resected, but until now the oedema phenonena has not happened. Headache, dizzy, pain of back, cardiac illness all are disappeared marvelly by exercising Guo Lin Qigong. The therapy of Guo Lin Qigong is fundamental therapy. It not only makes me recovered my health, but also gives me benefits in spirit and psychology. Through the exercises of Qigong my spirit is joyful, my heart is open and light, my ideology is clear. Guo Lin Qigong is one indispensable part of my life.

My western medical doctor also appreciated deeply the effect of my exercises with Guo Lin Qigong.

Case 2

Name: K. B. Sex: M. Bayer, Germany

Illness: Myelogenous Leukemia

Follows are the speech in the First Guo Lin Qigong World Congress (Bad Münstereifel, Germany 26-28, Sept, 2008)

Dear Madam Li WANG, Köln Guo Lin Qigong Akademie,

In this congress I would like to introduce my illness situation and the results after exercising Guo Lin Qigong.

In the routine health test of 2004, the CML Myelogenous Leukemia was diagnosed out from my body. This is a rare cancer of leukemia. Only until the beginning of 2000 there had been drug for therapy. But this drug is not affected for any person. Then with the recommendation of my physiatrist, I took part in the Guo Lin Qigong course organized by Am Steigenwald TCM Klinik two times. At the same time of therapy of drugs, I exercised Guo Lin Qigong. At the beginning my movement was not controlled with programs. With the supervision and guiding of Prof. Li Wang, I regulated my exercise gradually better and better. Every day I did the exercises one hour (every action I used to do 5-6 times). The contents of exercises are including **"Wind Breath", "Natural Go"** and **"Ascending, Descending, Opening and Closing"**. The Qigong exercises increased my immunity and healthy. The most importance was the blood laboratory test reached normal values. The Qigong movements has made me harmony and balance in my spirit. This is also very important. After 2 months' exercises continually, I recovered my work and can competent every kinds of tasks.

Follows give an interested example in exercise. In exercising the "Natural Go" I swing my double hands according the principle of "palm towards down", with not a long time, the index of the haemoglobin had been reduced. At the direction of Master Li Wang, I changed to "palm towards up", and then my blood index of haemoglobin had been ascended. I must emphasize in this period of exchanging direction of palms, my dosage of western medical drug and Qigong exercises are same as before absolutely. So, I could control and regulate my postures and movements to suit my symptoms very skilfully.

I extend cordial greetings for this congress successfully. I also would like to take place for your courses in the future.

K. B. Bayer, Germany

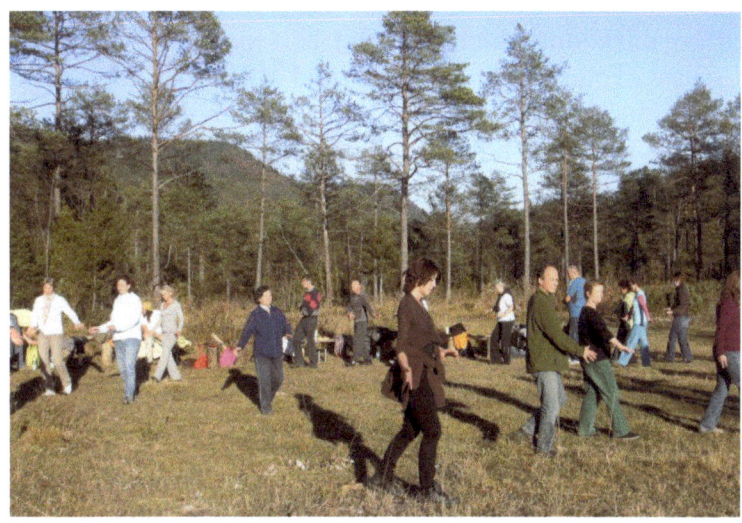

Fig.28 Guo Lin Qigong in Alpen Germany

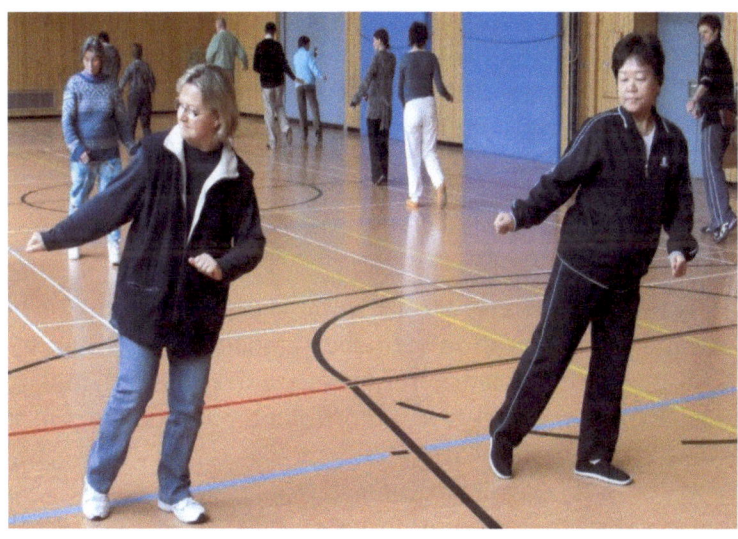

Fig.29 Ms.Maldener exercises Guo Lin Qigong under the supervision of Master Li WANG

5. Chinese Medicine is Holism Medicine

The Holism is unification and Integration. Chinese medicine pay attention to the holism of human body. The human body is a unified organization, which may not be separated. All the organs and tissues of the body regulate and affect to each other in physiology, and influence to each other in pathology. On the other hand, human is a same holism with the nature. Humankind must be suitable with the natural environment. These two sides compose the holism of Chinese medicine. This holism runs through all the physiology, pathology, diagnosis, differentiation, therapy and rehabilitation in Chinese medicine.

Five Organs (Liver, heart, lungs, spleen and kidney) are the centre of human body, which accompany with Six Fu (Gallbladder, small intestine, stomach, large intestine, bladder and San Jiao), and connect the four limbs, brain, bone, muscle, skin by Jing Luo (meridian). All the organs and tissues compose a complete holism. The body fulfils all functional activities with the good capabilities of Qi, blood, essence and fluid.

Human body is composed by organs and tissues, every organ has self function, but they have closed relation to each other. For example, a patient suffers from stomach illness, Chinese doctors don't pay attention to which bacteria or virus in stomach, they analyse syndromes of digest system (spleen and stomach, etc.) of the patient and their Yin and Yang balance. At same time they analyse the relation between spleen, stomach and other organs, **especially with liver, etc.** Of cause they also pay attention of the food, drinking and **emotion** (whether damaged and stimulated?), and the influence of weather (especially for **cold and moisture**). On the base of above analyses and differentiation, doctor can treat with recipe.

The above is the program of **diagnosis of TCM — "Wàng", "Wēn", "Wèn", "Qiè".** "Wàng" (望) is inspection: face colour, eye, skin, hair, **tongue and coating**, action and movement, etc., "Wēn"

(闻) is listening and smelling, "Wèn" (问) is inquire: syndroms, case history, "Qiè" (切) is **pulse** of radial artery. After diagnosis doctor makes differentiation, and therapeutic proposal are offered.

The heart is considered to be the most important organ of the body by TCM, the activities of lungs, spleen, liver and kidney all are based on the heart. The heart opens on tongue. So, when we observe the situation of tongue and coating, the physiology and pathology of patient could be realized. **The diagnosis of tongue and pules are important methods of TCM.**

5.1. The Principle of Yin-Yang is Differential Medicine

Chinese ancient thinkers had discovered all the phenomena and objects have the two sides of front and reverse, e.g. day and night, exposed and back to sun, active and silent, cold and warm, dry and moist, disease and healthy, etc. These phenomena and objects were abstracted as concept of "Yin 阴" and "Yang 阳" to explain the pattern of two kinds of opposite things which growth and decline to each other as well as their developmental law in the nature.

For the human body, Wu Zang (五脏 Five Organs) is Yin and Liu Fu (六腑 Six Fu) is Yang; the energy (Qi 气) is Yang and the substances (Blood, fluid) are Yin; the back of body is Yang and abdomen is Yin; the function of organs (digest, catharsis, storage, Qi transformation) is Yang and the tissue of organ is Yin. For Nature, wind, heat and dry are Yang; cold, moisture is Yin.

5.1.1 Basic Contents of Yin-Yang Principle

Lao Zi (老子 B.C. 577- ?, Great Philosopher, author of 《 Dao De Jing 道德经》 Fig. 30) pointed, "All objects are loaded by Yin and hold Yang in the cosmos", which means every thing is composed by Yin— substance and is given Yang— energy.

69

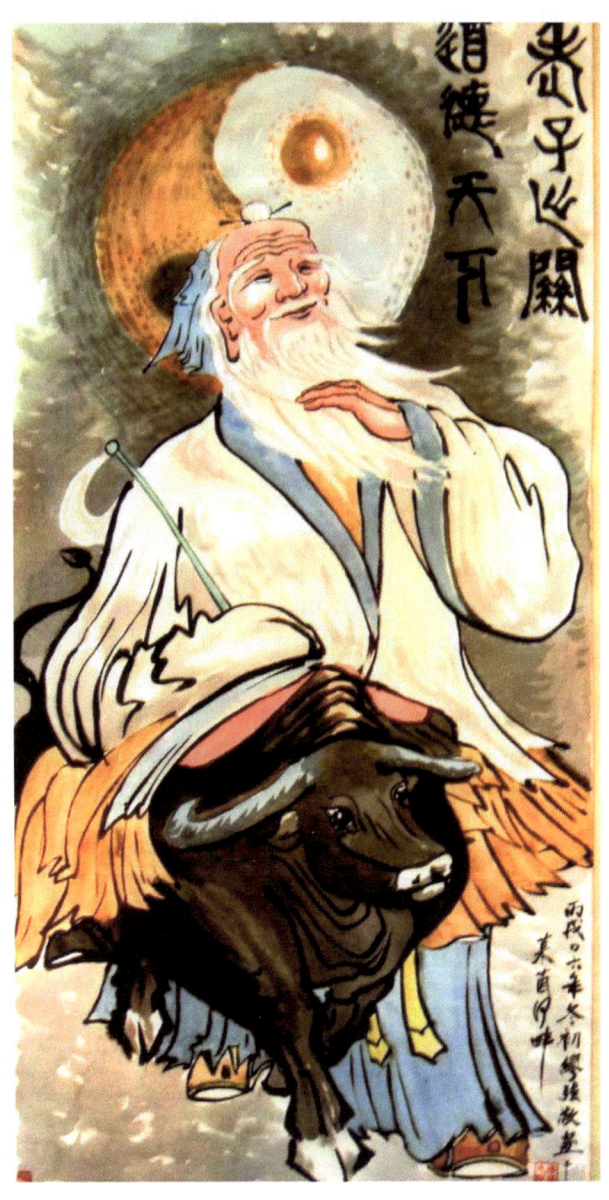

Fig. 30 Lao Zi

This illustrates either the relation between every object, and the law of unificate of opposite in the interior of one object.

The Principle of Yin-Yang is composed by the follows four parts:

5.1.1.1. Opposite and Restrict of Yin-Yang

There are dual character of opposite and restrict of all objects in the world, e.g. day and night, cold and warm, ascending and descending, light and dark, fire and water, etc.. This dual character maintains objects the dynamic balance, and promotes object to develop to the adverse direction, for example day alternates with night, change between cloudy and fine days, cold and warm days, etc. The growth and decline between two opposite sides make objects development, the nature could ever exist.

5.1.1.2. Interdependent

Yin and Yang is either opposite or interdependent. Yang takes charge of awakening and Yin is responsible growing, Yang controls ascending, developing and Yin controls storage, Yang masters Qi transform and Yin masters forming. Yin and Yang exist in an unifying system of restricting and changing, which have the mutual roots and existence. If there is not Yang, Yin will be disappeared; and if no Yin, Yang also can not existed.

5.1.1.3. Dynamic Balance

The balance of Yin-Yang is not static and absolute, only within a period and within a limitation Yin and Yang maintain a dynamic balance: sometimes Yin grows and Yang declines, or sometimes Yang grows and Yin declines. TCM calls this dynamics balance "Yang proper and Yin storage".

5.1.1.4. The Mutual Transform of Yin-Yang

In an exact condition, Yin and Yang will mutual transform towards opposite sides.

For example, one patient falls ill of acute infective hepatitis, the colour of skin and eyes became yellow, GOT and TTT, etc. of laboratory tests are not in normal. These mean the function of liver or/and other organs is with problems, in TCM this problem belongs "Yang" problem, which is "hyperactivity of liver-Yang".

If the therapy is not in time, propagating non-healing, after several months the acute hepatitis transformed to chronic hepatitis or hepatocirrhose. The follows syndromes are appeared: pain in chest, tired of body, poor appetite, watery and thin stool. These syndromes mean that tissues of organs (liver, spleen, stomach) have pathological changes, not only the function problem. This is the problem of Yin, i.e. "Yin deficiency". The above example illustrates in an exact condition "Yang syndroms" could transform to "Yin syndroms".

The TCM doctors observe the syndroms of Yin-Yang changing and their growing and declining in physiology and pathology of the patients at every time, and make different proposals of therapy.

5.2. Five Elements is Holism Medicine

Five Elements (Wu Xing 五行) are the motions of five elements (metal, wood, water, fire and earth). The ancient Chinese people thought all objects of the world were born by the motion and change between the five elements. This old philosophy concept, same as the Yin-Yang principle, has been contributed for the formation and development of TCM with far-reaching historical significance. (Fig.31)

5.2.1. The Characteristic of Five Elements

Except five substances, Five Elements also mean widely senses.

"Mu, 木 Wood" indicates the pattern of flora, also expresses growing, lifting, ascending, extending and catharsis.

"Huo, 火 Fire" indicates the pattern of burn, also expresses warm, heating, raising, energy.

"Tu, 土 Earth" indicates the pattern of soil, also expresses digesting, loading, accepting, base.

"Jin, 金 Metal" indicates the pattern of metal, also expresses cleaning, descending, astringent, transform, evolution.

"Shui, 水 Water" indicates the pattern of fluid, also expresses moistening, nutritious, down, cold, storage.

5.2.2. The Derivation of Five Elements

The principle of Five Elements derivates and classifies the characters of all the objects in the world based on the five substances' motion. The following table is the classification of the five elements characters of some other objects in human body and nature.

Five Tones	Jiao	Zheng	Gong	Shang	Yü
Five Tastes	Sour	Bitter	sweet	Pungent	Salty
Five Colors	Green	Red	Yellow	White	Black
Five weather	Wind	Heat	Moist	Dry	Cold
Five Changes	Living	Growing	Transform	Harvest	Storage
Five Direction	East	South	Center	West	North
Five Seasons	Spring	Sommer	Long Sommer	Autumn	Winter
五行 WU XING	木 Mu (Wood)	火 Huo (Fire)	土 Tu (Earth)	金 Jin (Metal)	水 Shui (Water)

Five Zang	Liver	Heart	Spleen	Lungs	Kidney
Liu Fu	Gallbladder	Small Intestine	Stomach	Large Intestine	Bladder
Five Sense Organs	Eyes	Tongue	Mouth	Nose	Ears
Five Tissues	Sinew	Blood Vessels	Muscle	Skin Fine Hair	Bone Hair
Five Emations	Anger	Joy	Worry	Anxiety	Fear
Five Voices	Call out Hu	langhter Xiao	Sound of singing Ge	Voice of cry Ku	Voice of chant Yin
Five Moves	Holding	Thinking	Tinkling	Coughing	Trembling

74

Five Elements

五　　行

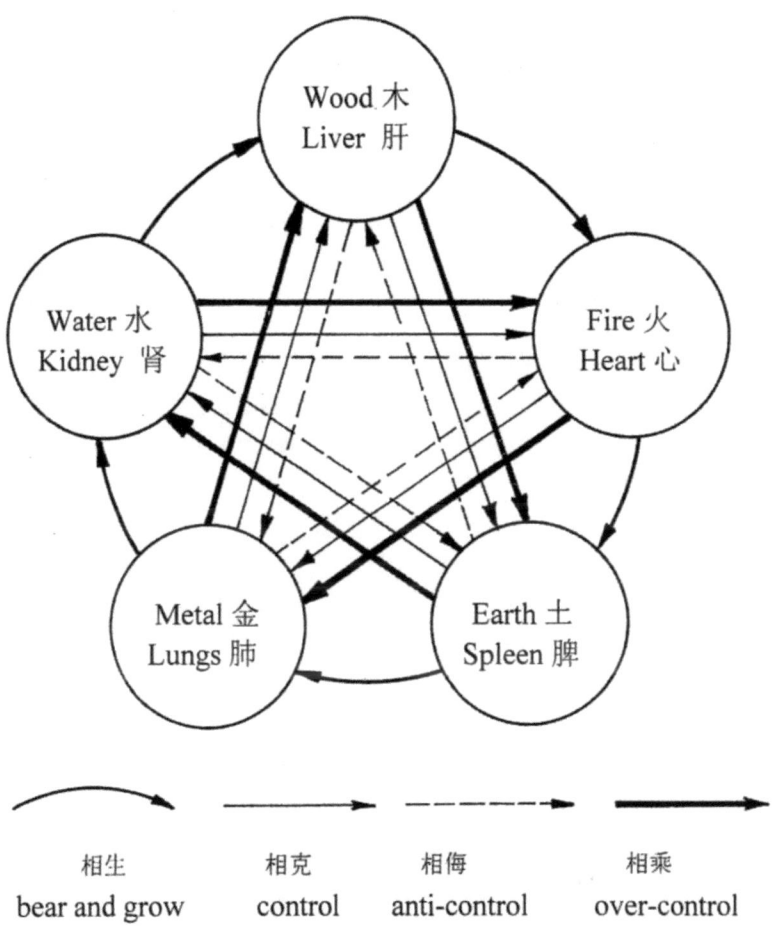

Fig 31 Five Elements

5.3 Chinese Medicine is System Science

When Chinese doctors differentiates the syndromes of patients, they always analyse and classify the syndromes into eight different kinds: exterior and interior; cold and heat; deficiency and excess; yin and yang. Except the organic differentiation, recently years some scholars put forward the Qi and Xue (blood) differentiation. In the same time Chinese doctors also take thinking about the human body is a huge-system, and every organ has relation to each other, they apply the principle of the "Five Xing" (five elements).

One important character of the **system science** is to classify the system into different **"situation"**. Chinese doctors just pay attention to this point, and therapy with differentiation for the syndromes. Because in different situation of human body, the different physiology reaction will be appeared to the aggression of "Liu Yin (6 kinds of

bad weathers); "Qi Qing (7 kinds of aggressive emotions) and the aggression of pestilences. For example, in the period of a raging pestilence broke out in one city, some person would be infected or dead, but much more other person were still healthy. This fact illustrates that different person has different situation, thereby they have different resistances for diseases. The famous bio-chemstrist prof. Linus Pauling (Nobel prize owner) used to said, "Orthomolecular to refer to the practice of varying the concentration of substances normally present in the body to prevent and treat disease".

The "Differentiation of Diagnosis" is means "To Look for Difference". After analyzing the "symptoms" of patients deeply and precisely, and getting the correct conclusion of the "Sydromes", doctors could make the exclusive and single-handed recipe of herbs; select the correct points and meridians for acupuncture to finish the therapy. This is the reason for "One patient, one recipe". Before 2000 years Chinese doctors had realized the concepts of

"Situation" and "Huge-System". This is also the essence of Chinese medicine.

The kinds of diseases could be reached about more than 30,000 according to modern medicine. In the ancient China the classification had been over 10.000 kinds. In this book the TCM therapy of hepatopathy is the main point which illustrates the differences between TCM and West Medicine in the fields of diagnose, analysis of cause and pathology, and the methods of therapy. At same time some important cases of illness and recipes by famous Chinese doctors including ancient and modern China are collected. These therapies have gotten good effect. In this book author analyses the principle of these therapy by the theory of bio-wave and cell molecular biology.

The chapter 6 expounds the physiological function of liver. The Chapters 7 and 8 discuss the therapies by herbs, and acupuncture for hepatosisis respectively.

5.4. Theory of Meridian is the Basis of TCM

《Shang Han Lun》(Treatise on the Colden Damage Diseases 伤寒论) was written by the famous TCM expert in Han dynasty by Dr.Zhang, Zhong Jing (张仲景 a.d.150-219) which is the first book for differential diagnose and therapy in China. Based on 《Huang Di Nei Jing》, 《Shang Han Lun》 established differential principle of 12 meridians. In diagnosis, West medicine pays attention to disease, but Chinese medicine takes care of the syndromes and patterns. There are 8 kinds of syndromes in TCM: Yin and Yang; exterior and interior; deficiency and excess; cold and heat. After diagnosing for the patient with the methods of "Wàng" (inspection 望), "Wēn" (listening and smelling 闻), "Wèn" (inquire 问), and "Qiè" (pulse 切), and realizing the patient's syndromes and physiological situation, Chinese doctors analyze differentially, and regulate Yin and Yang of the patient, then take the treatment.

Jing Luo is not same with the relevant organ. For example, the Jing Luo of liver is a meridian which begins from foot, leg, around the genital organ, and up to liver, head, eyes, finally arrives into brain (Fig. 32). The function of liver meridian is not only the digestion but also the catharsis, ascending Qi and storing blood, as well as controlling emotion. Combining the differential principle of Jing Luo and the five-element principle, paying attention to the function of self regulation and self repairing，TCM doctors could make the therapies more effective and with less side effects. The differential principle in TCM is one of the most important characters of the holism medicine. **The therapeutic recipe of TCM is based on syndromes; West medicine is based on disease. This is the difference between Chinese and West medicines.**

In the differentiation of TCM, the concept of "Qi" is very important. There are 4 kinds of "Qi": The first is "Yuan Qi", which is inborn and given from parents. The second is "Zong Qi", the oxygen from breath. The third is "Ying Qi", the nutrition and water. The fourth is "Wei Qi", resistance of evil Qi of outside. The movement of the 4 kinds of Qi will be realized by Meridian. The outside Qi which injures human body is called "Evil Qi". In next chapter we'll illustrate the "Liu Yin (Six Excesses)" and Pestilence, which all are belongs to "Evil Qi". The evil Qi injures into the body also from meridian.

5.5. The Cause and Pathogenesis of TCM

About the disease cause and pathogenesis, Dr. Zhang Zhong Jing appointed, "First is interior pathogenic Qi invade meridian and into organs, this is the inner cause. Second is harassment by exterior pathogenic Qi, the blood vessels which connect the four limbs and nine sense organs are blocked. And third is environment, trauma and pests". In Song dynasty (a.d. 960-1179) Dr. Zhang Wu Ze (张无择) according 《Jin Kui Yao Lue 金匮要略》 appointed, "The pathogeny has three causes: 6 Excesses (六淫 wind, cold, Sommer heat, moist, heat, dry), 7 Emotions (七情 joy, angry, anxiety, thought, grieved, frightened) and the Epidemic （疫疠.fear).

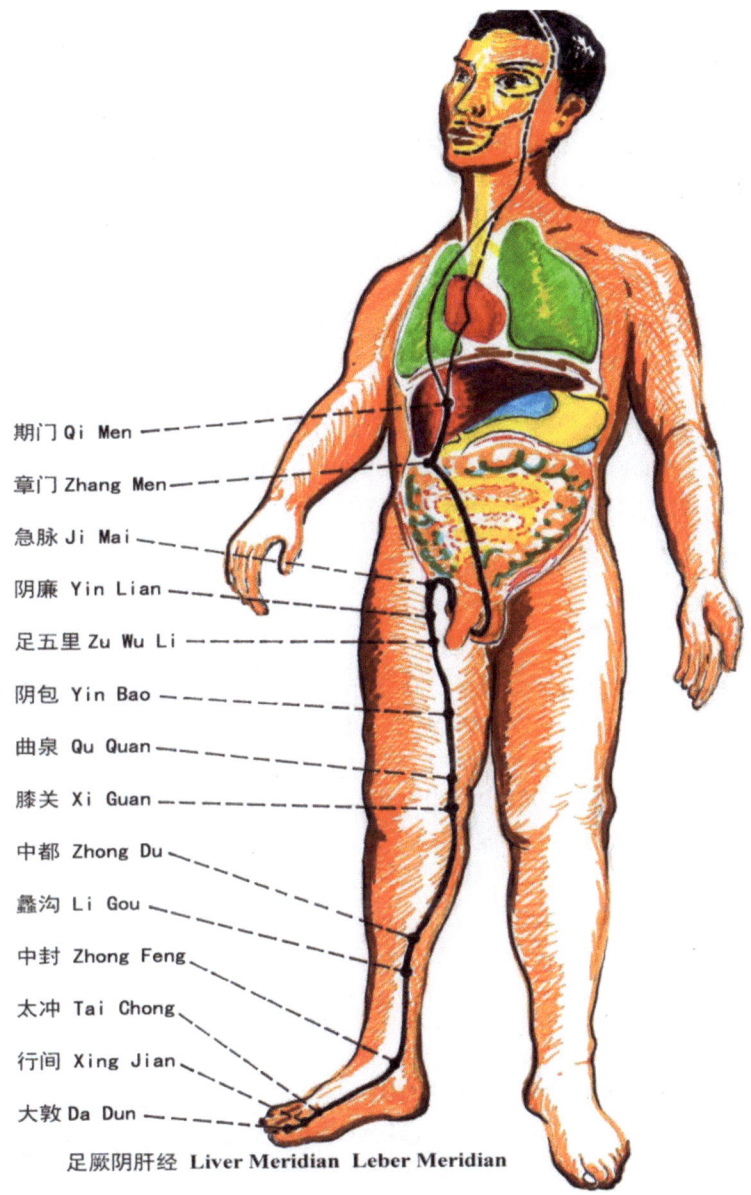

期门 Qi Men
章门 Zhang Men
急脉 Ji Mai
阴廉 Yin Lian
足五里 Zu Wu Li
阴包 Yin Bao
曲泉 Qu Quan
膝关 Xi Guan
中都 Zhong Du
蠡沟 Li Gou
中封 Zhong Feng
太冲 Tai Chong
行间 Xing Jian
大敦 Da Dun

足厥阴肝经 Liver Meridian Leber Meridian

Fig. 32 Liver Meridian

79

The above three causes lead to the conduction of bio-wave are resisted and blocked in meridian. At first the 3 Yang meridian (Hand-Yangming-Large Intestine meridian, Foot-Yangming-Stomach Meridian and Foot-Taiyang-Bladder Meridian) are damaged, then the 4 Ying meridian (Hand-Taiyin-Lungs Meridian, Foot-Jueyin-Liver Meridian, foot-Shaoyin-Kidney Meridian and Hand-Shaoyin-Heart Meridian) are brokendown. The blocked bio-wave makes the material transfer between micro-circulation and membrane of cell and the metabolic of cell are injured. At same time the transfer of electric signal and transmitters between nervous system and cell, as well as the exchange between endocrine glands of internal secretion and cell membrane also are influenced. At least the different diseases would be appeared in the human body.

TCM recognizes "Phlegm resists meridian". In TCM "Phlegm" means the waste produced after metabolism in the body and is not cleared away. In the Chapter 0.1 we know the velocity **V** of bio-wave is

$$\mathbf{V} = (\mathbf{G} / \, \rho \,)^{\frac{1}{2}}$$

G is the shearing model (Pa), ρ is the density (kg / cu.M). Due to the shearing model of phlegm is much lower than the tissues of body, the velocity of bio-wave is slow down, and the energy of the wave would be absorbed by phlegm. Thus, the meridian is blocked.

The above 3 causes of pathogeny all can induce the block of meridian, and the diseases will be happened from surface into the inner body.

Chinese medicine maintains, "there are not the syndrome which has no causes." To analyze the syndromes and physical signs of patients, and examine the diseases' causes, doctors could supply the foundation for therapy. In TCM these methods are called "to inquire the cause with differentiation." So, in diagnosis and cure, TCM pays attention to the "Syndrom", West Medicine pays attention to "Disease".

5.5.1. Six Excesses

Six Excesses are 6 kinds of evil pathogenic Qi: wind, cold, Sommer heat, moisture, heat, dry, which are the different whether of nature. If man could not adapt with the changing of whether, his meridian would be blocked and will be ill.

5.5.1.1. Wind

Wind always appears in spring season. Wind is YANG evil pathogeny, with character of opening, catharsis, towards up, exterior. Wind always invades YANG location of body, such as head, back, and muscle and Yang Meridian areas. The syndromes are headache, sweat, aversion to wind, the pulse is floating and tensive.

On the other hand, wind is easy to change and to run every where in the body, it can induce symptoms in different areas in the body, such as in head, skin, joints and liver. The diseases caused by invasion of wind are fast and urgent.

Wind is the No. 1 element of pathogenic. 《Huang Di Nei Jing》 said, "wind is the first cause of hundred illness." The pathogenis of cold, heat, moist and dry always invade body with wind, and the follows syndromes of illness will be appeared, such as rheumatic, wind-cold and wind-heat diseases, etc.

5.5.1.2. Cold

Cold is the pathogenic Qi in winter season. Cold is YIN evil pathogeny and always injures the Yang Qi of body. If cold invades body surface, the Meridian of "Hand Shao Yin Lung" would be damaged, and the follows syndromes are appeared: cough, common cold, sweat free. If cold invades spleen and stomach, and damages Meridian of Tai Yin Spleen, vomit, diarrhea will be happened. If cold wind invades heart and kidney, and Meridian of Hand Shao Yin Heart and Meridian of Foot Shao Yin Kidney damaged, the follows syndromes appeared: reversal cold of limbs, listless, dispirited.

The character of cold is stagnate and move sluggishly, and always make the Qi and Blood blocked, so the ache and pain will be appeared. 《Su Wen, one chapter of <Huang Di Nei Jing>》 said, "pain owing to cold," "ache due to cold stagnated." Cold makes meridian, muscle, skin and sinews systole, and pulse into custody, bend and stretch of body and limbs not freely.

5.5.1.3. Sommer-Heat

Sommer-heat is the Qi of summer season. Somme-heat is Yang evil Pathogeny, its character is blazing hot. It can make man with high fever, red face, perturb of heart and surging pulse.

Pathogenic Somme-heat consumes body's Qi and fluids, so symptoms are grand sweats, thirsty, red and short urine, sometimes due to deficiency of Qi, swoon appeared.

In summer season it is blazing hot, more raining, so the whether is hot with moist. The people always have the syndromes of vomit, breast sealed and diarrhea.

5.5.1.4. Moisture

The pathogenic moisture appears in summer and autumn seasons. Moisture divides the exterior moisture and the interior moisture. Exterior moisture is from whether. Interior moisture appears by the non-regulation of spleen & digest organ. The character of moist evil pathogenesis is heavy, and be detained in meridian and joints, the follows syndromes are appeared: headache, limbs weakness, body heavy. On the other hand, pathogenic moisture is filthy and increases secretions, the follows syndromes appeared: stool with blood and pus, urine not clear, skin ulcer, eczema and leucorrhoea for women.

Moisture is Yin pathogenic and blocks meridians, Qi and blood. Generally speaking, spleen organ likes dry and detests moisture. When spleen is invaded by moisture, its capability would be damaged, water and moisture are blocked in the body, ascites and water oedema would be appeared.

The Moisture pathogenesis and the waste of secretion are sticky. The illness caused by moisture always delay for a long time, such as liver cirrhosis, eczema, arthralgia, damp-warm diseases. The moisture pathogenesis likes running down in body, sometimes the following illness appear, ischuria, stranguria, leukorrhea, etc.

5.5.1.5. Dry

Dryness is the main evil Qi of autumn. In the beginning of autumn, the diseases appear owing to dry and heat. In autumn season it's colder day by day. In the later autumn the diseases happen due to cold and dry. The dryness pathogenic Qi always enters in the mouth and nose of men through the Meridian of Hand Tai Yin Lung, and invades windpipe and lungs.

The dryness pathogenic Qi consumes body fluids. The body loses Yin fluids and appears the syndromes of dryness of total body. The lung likes humid and moist environment, the dry pathogenic Qi damages lung easily. The lung controls breath, skin and fine hair, and opens on nose. The dryness pathogenic Qi lungs' decreases capability of dispersing up and descending down, the breath system diseases will be appeared.

5.5.1.6. Heat

The heat pathogenic evil Qi divides into two kinds: exterior heat and interior heat. The exterior heat is induced by Six Excesses, such as wind-heat, summer heat, and moist heat. The interior heat is produced by heart heat, liver heat and gallbladder heat.

The heat pathogenic Qi is Yang evil Qi, its character is towards up. The follows syndromes always happened: high fever, sweat out, perturbation, mania, delirious. The pulse is grand and quickly. The heat pathogenic Qi consumes Qi and fluids of body, makes people weak and exhaustion of body energy. It also produces "interior wind" which invades body to burn liver, consumes fluids, and loses nutrition for sinews. When "liver-wind" moves interiorly, the following syndromes appear: limbs twitch, spirit perturbed, delirious, neck unyielding.

The heat pathogenic Qi makes blood circulation flows violently, burns vessels, some hemorrhages appears: hematemesis, epistexis, hematochezia, hematuria, hemorrhage from skin, menorrheal and metrorrhagia for women.

The heat pathogenic Qi induces swollen sores. 《Ling Shu, another chapter of <Huang Di Nei Jing>》said， "Grand heat (fire) makes muscle putrefaction and saprophytism of pustule and sore which name is called carbuncles."

The heart controls blood circulation, and stores spirits, when heat pathogenic Qi invades heart the coma and obnubilation will be appeared.

5.5.2. Seven Emotions

"Seven Emotion" is seven kinds of emotions: over-joy, anger, anxiety, over-thinking, grieved, fear, frightened, which are the situation of spirits of mankind. Suddenly, strongly or continuously stimulating of emotions make people's Qi mechanism violent and chaos, meridian blocked, Qi and blood non-regulated, Yin and Yang unbalance, and organ injured with diseases.

Seven emotion is not same with Six Excesses. Six Excesses invade the organs of body from outside, but seven emotions injure organs from interior of body directly. The Five Organs produce Five Qi, the essences of five organs are the substantial Basis of the movements of emotion. The emotions of five organs are: heart with joy, liver with anger, spleen with over thinking, lungs with anxiety (grieved), kidney with fear (frightened). When the emotion's movement is excessively, the corresponding organ will be injured.

Seven emotions injure heart, liver and spleen more seriously than other organs. Heart controls blood and stores spirit, liver controls catharsis and stores blood. Spleen controls digest and locates in Middle JIAO (中焦), which is the hub of Qi mechanism. Spleen is the resources of Qi and blood. The dieses of heart, liver and spleen are closed with losing regulation of Qi and blood usually. 《Huang

Di Nei Jing 黄帝内经》said: "Anger injuring liver." To be the example, when man suddenly gets angry, the Qi and blood run towards up reversely and strongly, the follows syndromes are happed: hypochondriac pain and stress, coma and obnubilation of head, apoplexy. When Qi and blood are blocked, there will be some syndromes appeared, such as sight not clear, swollen and pain of liver and spleen, water and moisture stopped in organs, Ascites, etc.

5.5.3. Pestilence

Except Six Excesses, Pestilence is also an exterior pathogenic evil Qi, which is with strongly infective pathogenic Qi. 《Su Wen》 said，"When Pestilence comes, much more people are infected, which hasn't relation with ages, and the symptoms are similar."
That means before 2500 years, Chinese doctors had discovered pestilence could be infected through air, mouth, and nose and the pestilence can make illness and death in a large field.

6. The Difference between Chinese a. West Medicine from Physiological Function of Liver

The organ of liver belongs to "Wood 木" in "Five Element 五行" of TCM, which has the function of movement and ascending of physiology of human body. The liver is located in the belly, under the diaphragm, and in the right hypochondriac mainly. Liver is the house of soul, is the synthesis of total sinews, and is the store of blood.

The liver opens at the eyes; liver regulates sinew; the brilliance of liver is shown at the fingernails; the emotion of anger is controlled by the liver; the body liquid of the liver is tear. The liver and the gallbladder are exterior-interior pattern to each other.

6.1. The Catharsis and Storage of Blood

《Huang Di Nei Jing》 pointed out: "The main physiological function of liver are catharsis and storing blood in the body.

6.1.1. Catharsis

The Chinese word of catharsis includes two characters: "Shu 疏" and "Xie 泄". The meaning of "Shu" is dredge; "Xie" is effluent, generation and transformation. Liver can regulate Qi and promote the movement of blood and liquid of total body. The catharsis function of liver is including following three fields:

6.1.1.1. Regulate and Conduct the Qi Mechanism

The Qi's Mechanism includes ascending (and descending), enter (and exit) and motion. Due to the physiological function of liver are movement and ascending, liver is very important for dredgement, conduction and generation of Qi. If the function of catharsis of liver is normal, the Qi-Mechanism is conductive, Qi and Blood is harmonic, meridian is unobstructed, and the function of organs is regular. On the other hand, if the catharsis function of liver is not normal, there would be two symptoms:

A. the liver's catharsis function reduces, the ascending of Qi is not enough, the conduction of Qi Mechanism is resisted, and then Qi is blocked, there will be follows symptoms: distending pain in hypochrondriac, breast and belly.

B. the ascending of liver is too strong, the descending of Qi has not enough time to follow down, and then the Qi of liver moves toward up, there will be following symptoms: distending pain of head and eyes, red face and eyes, always anger. Due to the ascending of Qi is too strong, the blood flows with Qi along opposite direction, there will be some symptoms: spitting out blood, haemorrhage (tooth, nose, etc.), cough with blood, as well as Qi syncope, which is caused by the symptom of adverse flowing of blood. 《Su Wen 素问》 said, "Grand anger leads to Qi of body finished, and make blood towards up, the men will be emotional syncope."

The movement of blood and the arrangement of body fluids all rely on the ascending and descending movement of Qi. When Qi is blocked, there are barriers for fluids arrangement, and then some phlegm, water etc. of products of pathology are produced. Then the core of phlegm also be produced which is due to the meridian blocked. At least cirrhosis appears and ascites in belly happens. Qi's block conducts barriers of flowing blood, blood stasis, abdominal mass and hematoma. For women there will be menstrual irregularities, dysmenorrhea and amenorrhea.

6.1.1.2. Regulation and Conduction of Emotion

From TCM principle, the activation of emotion of mankind is the physiological function of the spirits controlled by heart. At same time, it also has the closed relation of the catharsis of liver. The fine emotion relys on normal movement of Qi and blood. When abnormal emotion appears Qi and Blood's movement will be disturbed. 《Su Wen》said, " hundred illness all are from Anger". When the catharsis function of liver is reduced, the Qi of liver will be blocked, and the state of mind is depressed. Oppositely when the ascending of liver Qi is too strong, the Yang Qi ascends toward up, the state of mind will be irritable. Even if having a not too big stimulation the anger will be appeared. Besides the manstructure and ovulation of women, the spermatogenesis of men all has closed relation with the catharsis function of liver.

6.1.1.3. Promote the Digestive Function of Spleen and Stomach

The digestive function of spleen and stomach depends on the harmony between the ascending of purity of spleen and the descending of filthy of stomach. If the catharsis function of liver is abnormal, the ascending function of spleen will be influenced: in the up direction, dizzy of head appears and in the down direction, diarrhea happened. At same time, when the function of descending mire of stomach damaged, the follows syndromes happen: vomit (on the up side), pain and expand of belly (in the middle area), and constipation (on the down side). IN TCM these are called "Qi of liver damages stomach" and "Qi of liver violates spleen". In the Principle of five Elements, this is meaning of "Strong wood attacks earth".

Liver and Gallbladder are exterior-interior to each other. The block of Qi of liver influences the secreting of bile and follows symptoms are appeared: distending pain in hypochondriac, bitter taste in mouth, digesting weakly, in special situation the jaundice happened. So 《Su Wen》 said," Earth is vitality after getting wood".

6.1.2. Store of Blood

Storing of blood of liver is meaning liver has the physiological function of storage of blood and regulation of volume of blood. Due to the blood belongs character of "Yin 阴", liver must store enough amount of blood, to control the ascending of the Qi (belongs Yang 阳), and maintains the Qi not too strong to protect the function of catharsis of liver. On the other hand, the storing of blood in liver can prevent haemorrhage in the human body. The third function of storing blood is liver can realize to regulate the blood volume in every parts of the human body, especially to protect the peripheral amount of blood. If the body's activity is intensively, or emotion is excited, the liver will distribute the stored blood outside arrangement to supply the requirement of relative organs. When man is in silence and maintains stable emotion, or in sleeping, much more blood will flow back into the liver again.

《Su Wen》said, "When man lies down, the blood returns back to liver".

Due to the function of storing and regulating of blood of liver, the physiological activities of every organs of the body have closed relation with liver. If the blood of liver is not enough, the eyes could not have enough nutrition, the symptoms of dry, poor vision and nyctalopia could be appeared. If the sinew can not get the nutrition from the blood, the follows symptoms will be happened: cramp of sinew, numb of body and four limbs, difficulty of bend and stretch of four limbs. For women, if liver blood is not enough, the hypomenorrhea and amenorrhea could be appeared; if the liver can not store blood, the hypermenorrhea, metrorrhagia and metrostaxis will be happened.

The function of regulating blood of liver is the balance between storing and catharsis of blood. If the function of storing blood reduces and catharsis increases, every kind of haemorrhage of body will happen; if liver is blocked and catharsis is weak, the blood stasis will happen.

6.2. The Relations between Liver and other Organs

According the principles of "Five Elements" and the theory of "Jing Luo", liver has closed relation with some other organs and tissues. The physiological situation of liver would influent the function of other organs and tissues directly.

6.2.1. Controlling Sinews in total Body

Sinews are the tissues connecting muscles and bones in whole body. The relaxation and systole of the sinews and muscles make the motion of the body. The sinews are dependent on the nutrition supplied by liver and blood. 《Ling Shu 》 appointed, "liver controls sinew", 《Su Wen》 said, "liver controls sinews and membranes of total body". If the Qi and blood of liver reduced and can't supply nutrition and sogginess to the sinews, the motion of the body will be tardy and not flexible. Sometimes the follows symptoms will be happed such as quiver of hand and foots, numb body, bending and stretching of the limbs not freely.

6.2.2. Making Brilliance of the Fingernails and Toenails

The fingernails and toenails are the continuation of the sinews. The prosperity or decline of the liver and blood influence the vitality or withered of the nails. If the liver blood is enough and abundant, the nails will be bright and tenacious. Oppositely when the liver blood is not enough, the nails will be not flat and firmly, with grey colour, and easy to split up and peel off.

6.2.3. Opening on Eyes

The meridian of liver connects up to the eyes. The vision of eyes relies on the nutrition of liver blood and the catharsis of liver. 《Su Wen》 said, "The eyes can be sense of sight only after accepted liver blood ." 《Ling Shu》 said, "The Qi of liver floats through eyes. It is depended on the harmony of liver that the five colors can be differentiated by eyes."

Chinese Medicine thinks about the essences of Five Zang (heart, lungs, spleen, liver and kidney) and Six Fu (Stomach, large and small intestines, gallbladder, bladder and San Jiao—thoracic cavity and abdominal cavity) all float and irrigate into the eyes. The eyes have closed relation with the total organs of the body. 《Ling Shu》 said, "the essences and Qi of Five Zang and Six Fu all flow to the eyes. The eye is the nestle of essence, the pupil is the essence of bone, the iris is the essence of sinew, the choroid is essence of blood, the sclera is the essence of nestle, the suspensorium ligament is the essence of muscle. The essences of sinew, bone, blood and Qi together with meridian float up to brain, and out from neck". (Fig. 33)

Because the relation between liver and eyes is very closed, it could be reflected by eyes that the function of liver is normal or not. If the liver YIN blood is not enough, the vision of eyes will be not clear and eyes feel dry. If the Liver-Wind removes interior, the limbs will quiver, the eyes will sight up. If the Liver-Fire runs up through the body, the eyes will be red color and swollen. If the Liver-Yang is extreme high, the giddy and dizzy will be appeared.

6.2.4. Controlling Tear

The tears have the abilities of moistening and protecting the eyes. In normal situation, the tears volume secreted not too much and not too small, and not spill over. But in the pathological situation the tears secreted unusually. If the liver blood is not enough, the two eyes sight objects not clearly and feel pain and dry. If the emotion is deeply grieved, tears like fountains welling up. If the meridian of liver is injured with wind and heat, the eyes will be red colour and swollen, or will tear when towards wind.

6.2.5. Hiding Soul

《Ling Shu 灵枢》 pointed out, "Soul is with coming and going of the spirit". The soul and the spirit all are on the substantial base of blood. The heart controls blood, so it stores spirit; liver stores blood, so soul can be hidden in liver. If the capability of storing blood of liver is in normal, the soul could hide there. If the liver blood is not sufficient, the follows phenomena would appear: more dreams, unstable, sleeping walking, and hallucinosis.

91

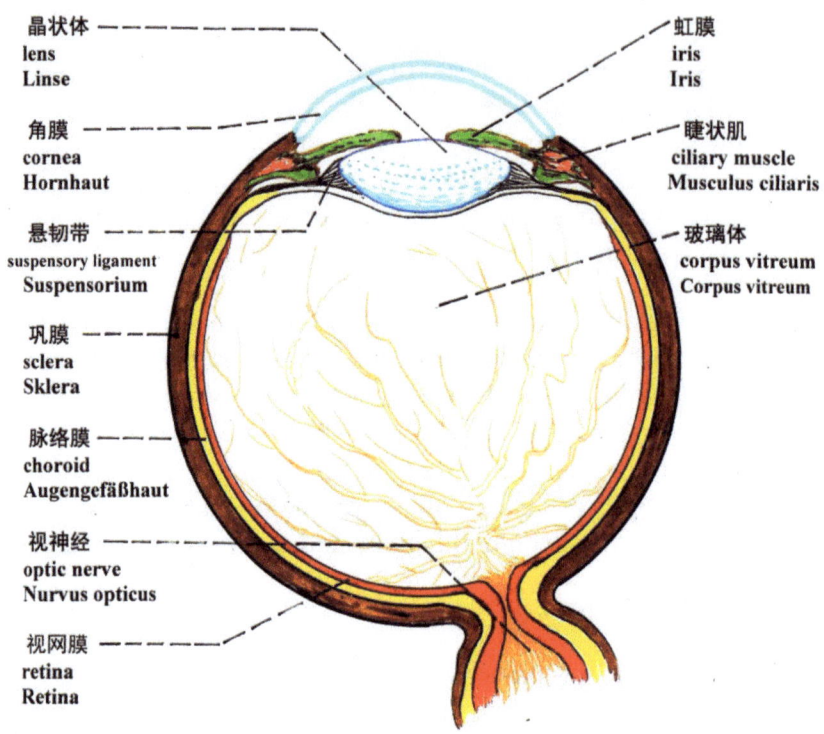

晶状体
lens
Linse

角膜
cornea
Hornhaut

悬韧带
suspensory ligament
Suspensorium

巩膜
sclera
Sklera

脉络膜
choroid
Augengefäßhaut

视神经
optic nerve
Nurvus opticus

视网膜
retina
Retina

虹膜
iris
Iris

睫状肌
ciliary muscle
Musculus ciliaris

玻璃体
corpus vitreum
Corpus vitreum

Fig. 33 Eye

7. The Differentiation and Herbs Therapy of Hepatopathies

Before 2000 years Dr. Zhang, Zhong Jing had classified the liver diseases to different kinds in detail in his works 《Shang Han Za Bing Lun 伤寒杂病论》.

	TCM	West Medicine
1	Yang Huang 阳黄	Acute Infective Icterohepatitis
2	Yin Huang 阴黄	Chronic Hepatitis
3	Ji Jü 积聚 Zheng 癥	Hepatocirrhose (with fixed gelosis)
4	Ji Jü 积聚 Jia 瘕	Hepatocirrhose (with moveble gelosis)
5	Shui Gu 水鼓	Ascites due to Cirrhose
6	Xue Gu 血鼓	Hepatocarcinoma
7	Ji Huang 急黄	Hepatonecrosis, Hepatic Coma

For the above different diseases Chinese medicine has had different diagnoses, differentiation and therapies respectively.

7.1. The Principle of Cellular Molecular Biology for the Cure of Chinese Herbs

The most important treatment of TCM is to regulate "Qi" and "Xue" of patient. In our research we found "Qi" is the bio-wave which conducts in Meridian. "Xue" means the micro-circulation and circulation of blood. Due to the action of bio-wave it's possible that the membrane could have active fluidity; Na^+-K^+ pumb can operate normally; membrane has enough resting potential, all of these guarantee the fine exchange of materials, energy and information between cell and micro-circulation. When person is ill, that means Qi and/or Xue meet with block, the membrane, plasma and nucleus have not normal physiological activities. In the more than 5000 years' history, many herbs were discovered to have the function for regulating "Qi" and "Xue" in China.

Why the Chinese herbs can cure illness? At first this is due to the "differential" principle in TCM. There are 8 different syndroms: Cold or Warm; Exterior or Interior; Deficiency or Excess and Yin or Yang. These eight different "states" show the four different non-balances situations. The usage of herbs can regulate the states and make the state reach balance. This theory is same with the physiologe of west medicine indeed. In 19 century famous France physiologist Prof. Claud Bernard (1813-1878) put forward the concept of "Homeostasis of inner Environment" He said:" The constant inner environment is the first condition of free and independent living for the body. All mechanisms of life only have one aim of maintaining inner environment stable, even if Prof.Linus Pauling (1901-1994) the kinds and function are different". In 1926 American physiologist Cannon WB (1871-1945) presented "Hemeostasis" concept. Hemeostasis is also called "Self-Hemeostasis", "Balance inner body" and "Constant Homeostasis".

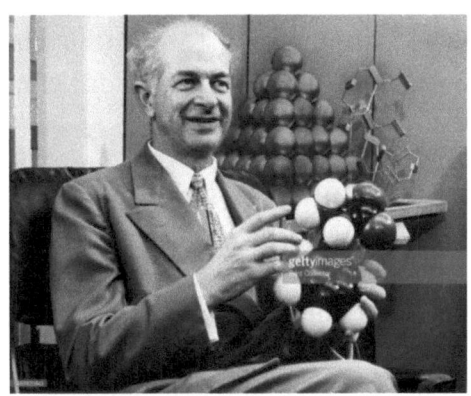

Fig.34 Prof. Linus Pauling

He considered variation is absolute and stable is relative, homeostasis is the process of regulating physiological activities from movement to silence. The famous American molecular chemist Prof. Linus Pauling (Fig.34) raised the concept "Correct Molecule" in 1954, he appointed, "the correct molecular medicine could prevent and cure disease through changing the different densities of every materials to reach balance in the body". Using of herbs is just for increasing the "Density of Correct Molecules". 1954 Nobel reisp owener.

At first some of the herbs have the function of increasing activity of membrane. For some serious illness, such as heart failure (owing to toxicosis, over tired) herb Huang Qi (黄芪 Radix Astragali Membranaceae Fig 36) could raise the resting potential of membrane, strengthen bio-wave, increase the fluidity of membrane and enhance "Qi", so the coronary artery and peripheral blood vessel of total body will be dilatated, the heart could recover function gradually. Under similar reason Huang Qi could increase the ratio of albumin for liver cirrhose, prevent ascites and decreasing of glycogen and recover the function of liver cell. Huang Qi can also delay the occurence of proteinuria and hypercholesterolemia. The experiments show that Huang Qi has function of delating coronary artery and capillaries; it has the fuction of reducing blood pressure BP. Bei Sha Shen (北沙参 Radix Glehniae Littoralis Fig.38), Dang Shen (党参 Radix Codonopsis Fig. 39), Bai Zhu (白术 Rhizoma Atractylodes Macrocephalae Fig. 40), Ginseng (人参 Radix Ginseng), etc. also have the function of enhancing Bio-Wave.

On the other hand, some of herbs such as Dang Gui (当归 Radix Angelicae Fig. 42), San Qi (三七 Radix Notoginseng), Chi Shao (赤芍 Radix Paeoniae Rubra) are very sensitive for "Xue" (hematopoiesis and circulation systems). Dang Gui could strengthen the function of hematopoiesis of spleen obviously, nourish blood and promote tissue regeneration; marvelously it has the double functions for menstruation illness: either exciting myometrium with its alkaloid (for therapy of menstrual disorder) or inhibiting and delaying myometrium with its content of essential oil (for therapy of metrorrhagia). It is same that San Qi has the functions of hematopoiesis and hemostasis.

The therapy of TCM could regulate one kind of state of patient to another state, from non- balance to balance. For example, to treatment fever, at first doctors of TCM must differentiate the state of patient: "Yin-Dificiency" or "Exterior-Excess". For the former, the disease means organic damage, usually uses herbs for nourishing Yin, invigorating Qi and Xue and uses a few purgative herbs; for the latter the illness means problem of function, usually uses herbs for relieving exterior evil syndrome and eliminating heat.

Through treatment patient could transfer from non-balance to balance and recovery.

TCM and West Medicine developed with two different ways: Meridian and Anatomy respectively. We hope the two medicines could be co-operated to find a more efficiency method for prevention and therapy of diseases on the basis of modern bio-physics, physiology and cellular molecular biology.

7.2 Acute Infective Icterohepatitis

Liver belongs of Wood in Five Elements. Spring season is the time of growing of plants. The infective icterohepatitis will be appeared in spring always. There are much more winds in spring. The character of wind is running and variable, if there is pestilence pathogenic Qi, the acute infective icterohepatitis will be epidemic. So, the incidence of acute infective icterohepatitis in spring season is more. This hepatopathies is divided to five kinds of A, B, C, D and E types. In TCM this disease is named "Yang Huang" (阳黄 Yang Yellow).

7.2.1. Disease Causes and Differentiation

There are two causes of this acute icterohepatitis, first is the exterior moisture and heat pathogenic evil invade body, Qi mechanism of body is resisted, the moisture and heat enter into blood, damage spleen and stomach, digest system is not running in order, liver loses the capability of catharsis. If in the same time there is virus with pestilence, the infective hepatopathies will spread. The second cause is inappropriate diet damages spleen and stomach, the pathogenic moisture and heat are produced in the interior organs themselves, Qi and Blood are blocked, and then liver and gallbladder are injured.

For more effective and accurate therapy, it is necessary to differentiate the syndromes of the patients of acute infective icterohepatitis. The differentiation could be diagnosed and analyzed as follows four situations.

7.2.1.1 Icteric and non-Icteric

Icteric Hepatitis	Serious moisture and heat	Moisture and heat not only resists Qi,but also blocks blood vessels, then toxy and phlegm are produced, make bile out of tube and bile enters into blood vessels over all the body. The icteric syndrome happens.
Non-Icteric Hepatitis	Light moisture And heat	Moisture and heat pathogenic evil only blocks Qi mechanism, not enters into blood, the bile can flow within normal tennels.

7.2.1.2. Moisture and Heat

	Diagnose	Differentiation and therapy
Serious moisture and Light heat	Pulse slippery and deep, white tongue coating, head and body feeling heavy, abdomen feeling distension, stool is watery and smashed.	Give priority to drain moisture and clearing heat auxiliary. The herbs of Yin Chen (Virgate Wormwood), Mu Dan Pi (Peony root bark), Da Huang (Rhubarb), etc. could be used
Serious heat and Light moisture	rapid and wiry pulse, tongue coating yellow, dysphoria, thirsty.	Give priority to clear heat and draining moisture auxiliary. The herbs of Yin Chen (Virgate Wormwood), Zhi Zi (treated Cape Jasmine Fruit), Bai Zi (Chinese Arborvitae Kernel), etc. could be used.

7.2.1.3. Deficiency and Excess

Excess Syndrome	Invasion period	In the invasion period of Acute Hepatopathies, course develops rapidly, the moisture and heat pathogenic evil Qi enter into body, capability of organs is imbalance. But in this time the body healthy Qi still exists even the pathogenic Qi is grand. Eliminating pathogenicity is the main side of therapy. The follows herbs could be adopted: Qing Hao (Sweet Wormwood), Yin Chen (Virgate Wormwood), Jin Qian Cao (Lysimachiae),
Deficiciency Syndrom or Excess plus Deficiency	Recovery Period	When above syndromes disappeared, the eliminating pathogenic herbs shoud be stopped using. In this time when using attacking and drastic formula herbs, herbs of reinforcing Body Qi and tonifying blood should also be used, such as: Gan Cao (Liqorice Root), Da Zao (Chinese Date), Bai Zhu (Atratylodis Rhizome), Bei Sha Shen (Coastal Glehnia Root), Mai Dong (Dwarf Lilyturf Tuber), etc. If patient is very strong and is with execess syndrome, it's not necessary to use tonic herbs.

7.2.1.4. Yang Icteric and Yin Icteric

	Invasion Time	Differentiation and Treatment
Yang Icteric (阳黄)	Beginning of Invasion	Pestilence invades Yang Ming L.I. and ST. Meridian, moisture and heat attack liver, the bile flows outside from vessels, and body with yellow colour. Eliminating moisture and heat pathogen is the main therapy principle.
Yin Icteric (阴黄)	With the history of hepatitis	The colour of face is black and shallow, the skin is yellow and sallow. Chronic hepatitis patient is at acute invasion period. The main therapy is using tonic herbs for body Qi and blood, and regulating fuction of spleen and stomach.

7.2.2. The Composition of Herbs Recipe

In recipe of Chinese herbs, the function for every herb is different. According the function of therapy, in a recipe the herbs are divided into four kinds:

"King Herb (君 Jun)", "Minister Herb (臣 Chen)", "Officer Herb(佐 Zuo)", "Ambassador Herb(使 Shi)". "Jun herb" is the most important herb which has key function for therapy. "Chen herb" is similar as Jun herb and enhances its function. "Zuo herb" is auxiliary herb, e. g. for acute hepatitis, the function of King and Minister herbs are eliminating moisture and heat, at same time some herbs for tonifying body Qi and blood are necessary, which are the "Zuo herbs". The function of "Shi herb" has tropism for referential meridians guiding the efficiency of herbs into the correspondent organs and tissues.

中文	PIN YIN	LATIN	English	German
茵陈	Yin Chen	Artemisiae Scopariae	Virgate Wormwood	Besenbeifuβ -kraut
草河车	Qi Ye Yi Zhi Hua	Phizoma Paridis	Paris Rizoma	Einbeerenwurzel -stock
金钱草	Jin Qian Cao	Herb Lysimachiae	Christina Loosestrife	Felbrich
金银花	Jin Yin Hua	Flos Lonicerae	Honeysuckie Flower	Geiβ blattblüten
橘红	Ju Hong	Exocarpium Citri Rubrum	Red Tangerine Peel	Rote Mandarinenschale
赤勺	Chi Shao	Paeoniae Rubrae	Red Peony Root	Pfingstrosenwurzel
泽兰	Ze Lan	Herb Lycopi Lucidi	Hirsute Shiny Bugleweed	Wolfstrappkraut
藿香	Huo Xiang	Herb Pogostemonis	Cablin Patchouli	Patchouli-Kraut
蒲公英	Pu Gong Ying	Herb Taraxaci	Dandelion	Löwenzahnkraut
生甘草	Sheng Gan Cao	Radix Glycyrrhizae Preperata	Liquorice Root	Ural-Süholzwurzel

This recipe is from Prof. Guan, You Bo, Beijing, China

King Herb: Yin Chen, Virgate Wormwood. (Fig. 35)

Flora: Composite family, Perennial, Seedling.

Character: bitter, middle.

Tropism to meridian: spleen, stomach, liver and gallbladder.

Function: Eliminate moisture and heat, clear away Icterus.

Component : P-hydroxyphenyl, volatile oil (β-pinene, capillin, folacin, alcoholate tujyl)

Pharmacology: P-hydroxyphenyl can increase the bile secrete, and enhance the output of solid, cholic acid and bilirubin from liver. Yin Chen has strong antipyretic function. Volatile oil has powerful inhibitate function for virus and bacteria. It can detoxicate for liver through urination.

KING HERB	PIN YIN	茵陈 YIN CHEN
君　药	LATIN	Herba Artemisiae Scopariae
	ENGLISH	Virgate Wormwood Herb
	GERMAN	Besenbeifußkraut

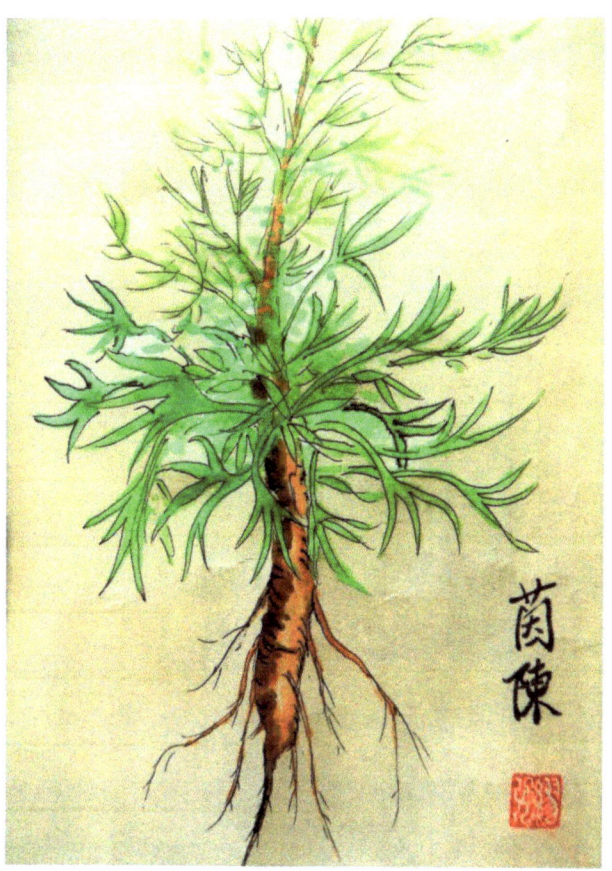

Fig. 35   Yin Chen

103

In differentiation of Acute Icterohepatitis, if the follows 12 obverious syndromes are seriously, it is possible to increase following different herbs respectively.

Obverious Syndrom	Plus Herbs	PIN YIN	LATIN	English	German
Heavy Moisture 湿重	佩兰 白术 薏苡仁 茯苓	Pei Lan Bai Zhu Zi Zi Ren Fu Ling	Eupatorii Fortunei Atractylodis Semen Coicis Sclerotium Poriae	Feverwort White Atractylodes Coix Seed Hoelen	Wasserdost Atractylodes Hiobstränensamen Kokospilz
Heavy Heat 热重	山栀 黄芩 黄连 大黄	Shan Zhi Huang Qin Huang Lian Da Huang	Gardeniae Jasminoidis Scutellariae Baicalensis Rhizoma Coptidis Rhizoma Rhei	Gardenia-Fruit Scute Coptis Rhubarb	Gardenienfrüchte Baikal-Helmwurzel Goldfadenwurzelstock Rubarbwurzel
Fever, Aversion to cold 发热恶寒	桑叶 生石膏	Sang Ye Sheng Shi Gao	Folium Mori Albae Gypsum	Mullberry leaf Gypsum	Maulbeerblätter Gips
Vomit 呕吐	生赭石 旋复花	Sheng Zhe Shi Fu Xuan Hua	Ochre Flos Inulae	Ochre ElecampaneFlower	Ochre Alantblütten
Chest Pain 两胁疼痛	柴胡 当归 白芍 香附	Chai Hu Dang Gui Bai Shao Xiang Fu	Bupleurum Angelicae Sinensis Paeoniae Lactiflorae Cyperi Rotundi	Bupleuri Tangkui Root White Peony Cyperus Rhizoma	Hasenohrwurzel Angelikawurzel Wei β pfingstrosen Nusswurzelstock
Stomach suffocated sealed 胃堵	木香 砂仁	Mu Xiang Sha Ren	SaussureaeLappae Fructussen Semen	Auklandia Grain-of-Paradis Fruit	Echtekostwurzel Amomumi-Sharen Früchte

Anorexia, Abdomen Distension 食欲不振腹胀	菜服子 焦三仙 厚补 白术 茯苓	Cai Fu Zi Jiao San Xian Hou Bu Bai Zhu Fu Ling	Semen Paphani Sativi Magnoliae Atratylodes Sclerotium Poriae Cocos	Radish Seed Burnt Bread Magnolia Bark WhiteAtractylodes Hoelen	Rettichsamen Verkohlt Brot Magnolienrinde Atractylodeswurzel Kokospilz
Heorrhage Epistaxis 出血衄血	白茅根 牡丹皮 藕节炭 大黄炭 阿胶	Bai Mao Gen Mu Dan Pi Ou Jie Tan Da Huang Tan E Jiao	ImperataeCylin dricae Cortex Moutan Radicis Nodus Nelumbinis Rhizoma Rhei Gelatinum Corii Asini	White Grass Peony Rootbark Lotus Rhizoma Node Burnt Rubarb Root Ass Skin Glue	Alang-Alang-Gras Strauchpaeonien Lotusrhizomanoten Verkohlt Rhabarber Eselshaut-Gelatine
Liver swollen spleen swollen Chest Pain 胁痛 Seriously 肝脾肿	生牡蛎 丹参 泽兰 红花子	Sheng Mu Li Dan Shen Ze Lan Hong Hua Zi	Concha Ostreae Salviae Miltiorrhizae Herb Lycopi Lucidi Carthami Tincorii	Oyster Shell Red Sage Root Bugleweed Safflower Seed	Austernschale Salvia-Wurzel Wolfstrappkraut Saflorblüten Same
Urine yellow and shaot 尿黄短 Urethra burn and pain_ 尿道烧痛	扁蓄 冬葵子 车前子	Bian Xü Dong Kui Zi Che Qian Zi	Polygoni Avicularis Semen Abutiliseu Malvae Semen Plantago Seed	Avicularis Malva Seed Plantago Seed	Vogelknöterichkraut Malvensamen Wegerichsamen
Abdomen pain, Diarrhea 腹痛痢疾 Anus burn and Pain 肛门烧痛	白头翁 葛根 黄芩 黄连 秦皮	Bai Tou Weng Ge Gen Huang Qin Huang Lian Qin Pi	Pulsatillae Chinesis Radix Puerariae Scutellaviae Baicalensis Rhizoma Coptidis Cortex Fraxini	Pulsatilla Root Kudzu Root Scute Coptis Ash Bark	Chin.Küchenschellen Kopoubohnenwurzel Baikal-Helmkrautwurzel Goldfadenwurzelstock Eschenvinde

Loins aching pain, Legs 腰酸 weakness 腿软	川续断 桑寄生 牛膝	Chuan Xu Duan Sang Ji Sheng Niu Xi	Dipsaci Asperi Ramulus Sangjisheng Achyranthis	Teasel Root Mulberry Mistletoestem Achyranthes	Chin.Kardenwurzel Riemenblume Achyranthis

**These recipes are from <The Analysis of Hepatisis Cases of Guan,You Bo> Page56 ZHAO Be ZhI, Beijing, China

7.2.3. Case

Mr. Feng, M. 17, student of middle school. 08, Feb. 1995 first visiting.

Syndromes: Icterus happened suddenly, skin and sclera all are yellow colour, dizzy, mouth bitter, urine red and yellow colour, stool dry, abdominal distension, vomit, anorexia, fever (37.4° C) afternoon, acratia.

Laboratory Report: GTP 2615, GOT 932, Alk. Phosphatase 193, GPT/ALAT 122, total bilirubin 138.51, bilirubin 83.79, Hepatitis A, antibody ImG positive.

West Diagnose: Acute Icterohepatitis.

TCM diagnose: Pulse: wiry, slippery and rapid. Tongue coating: white with yellow colour and thick, greasy.

TCM disease: Ji Huang, 急黄.

Differentiation: Pathogenic moisture and heat entering into organs, damping liver and gallbladder, resisting catharsis and pressing bile outside.

Therapy Principle: catharsis the blocked Qi of liver and gallbladder, clear away heat, remove moisture and detoxify.

The recipe of herbs

中文	PIN YIN	LATIN	ENGLISH	GERMAN	Dosage, g
茵陈	Yin Chen	Artemisiae Yinchen	Wormwood	Besenbeifuß	30
柴胡	Chai Hu	Radix Bupleuri	Thorowax Root	Chin. Hasenohrwurzel	14
黄芩	Huang Qin	Scutellaviae Baicalensis	Scute	Baikal-Helmkraut	10
栀子	Zhi Zi	Gardeniae Jasminoidis	Treated Gardenia	Verarbeitet Gardenien	10
仓术	Cang Shu	Rhizoma Atractylodis	Atractylodes	Mastixdistel	10
厚补	Hou Bu	Magnoliae Bark	Magnolie Bark	Magnolien Schale	15
陈皮	Chen Pi	Reticulatae	Tangerine Peel	Mandarinen Schale	10
法半夏	Fa Ban Xia	Pinillae Ternatae	Prepared Pinillia	Vorbehandelte Pinellia	12
竹茹	Zhi Ru	Bamboo in Taeniis	Bamboo Shavings	Bambusrohr Kraut	15
凤尾草	Feng Wei Cao	Herba Pterii	Pteris	Saumfarn Kraut	15
红花子	Hong Hua Zi	Carthami Tinctorii	Safflower	Saflorblüten	10

The patient took 7 doses of juices from the decocted herbs as above recipe. The Icterus colour has become shallow, vomit was reduced, body temperature also fell down. But the patient was still tired and acratia, urine with yellow colour, tongue with white and greasy coating, pulse is wiry and slippery.

The second recipe as follows:

中文	PIN YIN	LATIN	ENGLISH	GERMAN	Doges, g
茵陈	Yin Chen	Artenisiae Yinchen	Wormwood	Besenbeifu β	30
大金钱草	Da Jin Qian Cao	Herb Lysimachiae	Cristina Loosestrife	Felberich	30
垂盆草	Chui Pen Cao	Sedi Sarmentosi	Stonecrop	Fetthenenkraut	15
白花蛇舌草	Bai Hua She She Cao	Oldenlandiae	Oldenlandia	Oldenlandia	15
柴胡	Chai Hu	Herb Bupleuri	Thorowax Root	Chin. Hasenohrwurzel	15
黄芩	Huang Qin	Scutellaviae	Scute	Baikal-Helmkraut	10
土茯苓	Tu Fu Ling	Smilacis	Glabrous Greenbrier	Stechwindenstock	15
凤尾草	Feng Wei Cao	Herba Ptevii	Pteris	Saumfarnkraut	15
草河车, 蚤休	Cao He Che Zao Xiu	Rhizoma Oaridis	Paridis Rhizome	Einbeerenwurzelstock	15
灸甘草	Jiu Gan Cao	Uralensis	Licorice Root	Ural-Süβholz	4
泽兰	Ze Lan	Lycopi Lucidi	Bugleweed	Wolfstrappkraut	10
茜草	Qian Cao	Rubiae Cordifoliae	Madder Root	Krappwurzel	10

After the patient continued to drink 7 doses juices of the second recipe, his appetite increased grandly, the physical strength built up, every day one time of stool, yellow colour all were disappeared from body. The patient pathocured.

The laboratory report: GPT 141, GOT 421, Alk. Phosphatase 99, total Protein 82, Albumin 46, Bilirubin 35.91, LDH (Lactic dehydrogenase) 132.

Then the second recipe was taken 14 doses again. The report was: GPT 24, GOT 23, Alk. Phosphatase 99, LDH 135, Total Protein 80, Albumin 46, Bilirubin negative. The patient had recovered health and returned back to school.

** This case and recipe are from Prof. Liu, Du Zhou, Beijing, China

7.3. Chronic Hepatitis

Most of chronic hepatitis is caused by curing not in time or a long delay in the period of acute hepatitis. It makes patients weak of body Qi, and the evil Qi of moisture and heat has not been cleared out of the body. The syndromes of chronic hepatitis are total body acratia, chest pain, abdominal distension, poor appetite. The tongue coating is thin and with white colour, the pulse is thready, faint, deep and slow. Most of the patients are in follows situation: sleep loss, morale instability, over tired, or over alcohol drinking. In TCM this disease's name is "Yin Huang" (阴黄 Yin Yellow).

Most of the chronic hepatitises are with the types of hepatitis B and C, a small amount is of hepatitis D and E. The prognosis of chronic hepatitis is unfavourable which could develop to hepatocirrhosis and hepatocarcinoma.

7.3.1. Causes and Differentiations

7.3.1.1. The causes of chronic hepatitis

Generally speaking there are four pathogenies for chronic hepatitis.

A. Weakness of body Qi After suffered acute hepatitis, patient has had not enough rest and good cured, the organs' capability is unregulated, the digesting function of spleen and stomach is fall off, the essence of postnatal is damaged, and Body Qi can not clear out the evil Qi. If there are overwork or/and stimulations of emotion, the illness will be delayed for a long time, the acute hepatisis becomes to chronic.

B. Blood deficiency Liver is the organ of storing blood, it needs the nutrition and irrigation of blood. Due to the hepatitis propagates non-healing, the kidney and liver became weakness gradually, body Qi and Blood are produced less, and the blood becomes deficiency.

C. **Blood blocked** 《**Huang Di Nei Jing**》 **said, "The body's Qi is the vanguard of blood, the blood is the basis of Body's Qi.".** When Body Qi is weak, the blood can not run forward, and then blood is blocked and becomes into block of stuffiness, the fresh and new blood could not be circulated.

D. **Moisture and heat evil detained** The moisture and heat has been not all removed away, there are still evil of moisture and heat detained in the body. The liver, kidney and spleen has been damaged in this long period. The exterior evil and interior weakness induce hepatitis propagating and non-healing.

7.3.1.2. The differentiation and cure of chronic hepatitis

The integrative differentiation is necessary for chronic hepatitis. Moisture and heat are the main symptoms. In treatment reinforcing body Qi is the principle, and removing evil moisture and heat is auxiliary. The reinforce is meaning to regulate liver, kidney and spleen, especially for spleen. Rreinforcing spleen can enhance the capability of hemopoiesis, blood is the base of Qi, **Qi will be abundant and strengthen the action of bio-wave, and thus the capability of the cells of liver will be enhanced function and also make the demaged cells transform to normal cells.** Removing out the evil Qi must pay attention to activating blood and cooling blood, clearing heat, dispelling phlegm and resolving

110

dampness. Owing to the differentiation is a very complete process of diagnose, the famous Chinese doctors have had deeply researched in every dynasties of past 2000 years continuously. The follows five kinds of the differentiations of chronic hepatitis could be referenced for readers.

A. Body Qi and blood deficiency totally

Syndrome: dizzy, giddy, pale face colour, acratia of total body, sparse and thin hair, chest pain, weak sweat more, urine weakly and thin, stool watery and mashed.

Diagnosis: tongue coating: thin and less with white colour, tongue texture: pale. Pulse: deep, week and thready, without force. If Yin is too weakness, tongue texture with micro-gaps and with red colour.

Differentiation: Spleen loses normal function of digest, blood produced not enough, Body Qi consumed with blood, and Qi and Blood all are weak.

Cure: invigorating spleen, supplementing Qi.

The recipe of herbs

中文	PIN YIN	LATIN	ENGLISH	GERMAN	Dosage,g
生黄芪	Huang Qi	Radix Astragali	Yellow Milk-Vetch	Astragalus	30
党参	Dang Shen	Pilosulae	Asiabell Root	Glockenwinden	10

白术	Bai Zhu	Rhizoma Macrocephalae Atractylodis	Largrhead White Atractylodes	Großköpftig Atractylodes	10
茯苓	Fu Ling	Sclerotium Poriae Cocos	Hoelen	Kokospilz	10
白芍	Bai Shao	Paeoniae Glutinosae	White Peony	Pfingstrosen	15
生地黄	Di Huang	Rehmanniae	Fresh Chi .Foxglove	Frische Rehmannia	10
当归	Dang Gui	Angelicae	Tang Guei	Chi. Angelika	10
川芎	Chuan Xiong	Chuanxiong	Sichuan Lovage	Mutterwurz	10
甘草	Gan Cao	Uralensis	Licorice Root	Ural-Süβholz	6

King Herb: Huang Qi, Radix Astragali (Fig. 36)

Flora: Bean Family, Perennial, Herbaceous

Character: Sweet, Some Warm

Meridian: Spleen, Lunge.

Function: Reinforcing Qi, lifting Yang

Component: Carbohydrote, phlegm, choline, amino acids.

Pharmacology: Huang Qi could increase the ratio of albumin for chronic hepatisis and liver cirrhose, prevent ascites and increase glycogen and recover the function of liver cell. Huang Qi has the capability of contraction for heart, especially for the exhausted heart owing to intoxitation and tiredness. It has the function of dilatation for coronary artery and peripheral vessels to refine circulation and nutrition of cells. At last it can inhibit urinal protein and high chcholesterin.

KING HERB 君 药	PIN YIN	黄芪 HUANG QI
	LATIN	Radix Astragali Membranaceae
	ENGLISH	Membranous Milkvetch
	GERMAN	Astragaluswurzel

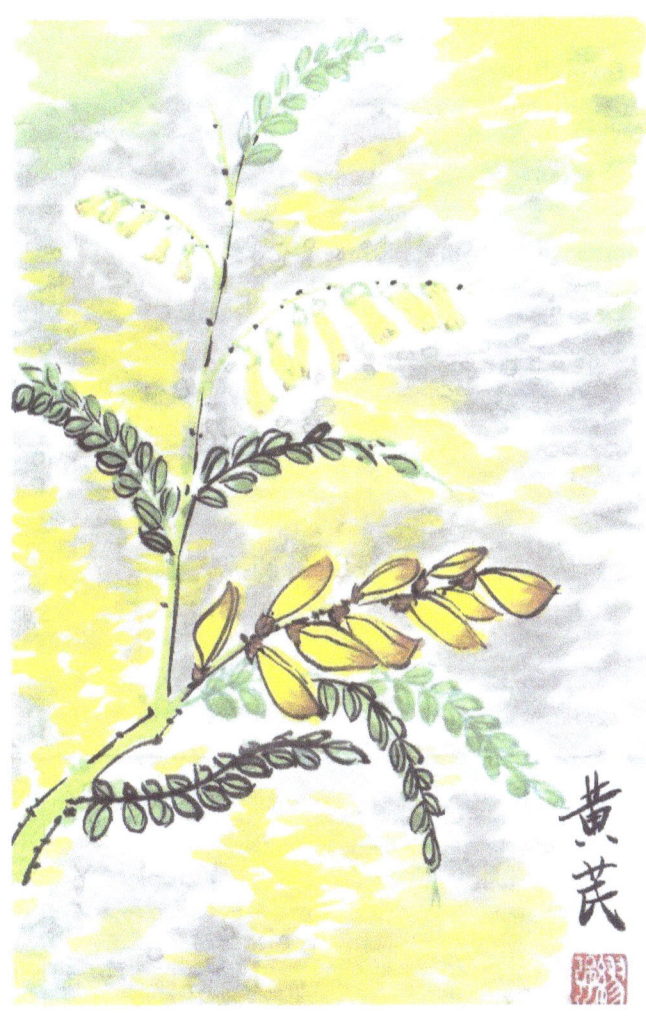

Fig. 36 Huang Qi

113

B. Liver and stomach harmonyless

Syndrome: vomit, stomach heartburn and acid regurgitation, pain in chest, abdominal distension.

Diagnose: tongue coating: white, pulse: wiry.

Differentiation: liver is "Wood" in "Five Elements", stomach is "Earth", wood controls earth, and Liver function strongly influences the function of stomach. Due to liver Qi is blocked, its conductive and catharsis function are weak, so stomach Qi is ascending adversely, the symptoms of vomit, heartburn, acid regurgitation and abdominal distension appear.

Cure: balance of liver and harmony of stomach.

The recipe of herbs

中文	PIN YIN	LATIN	ENGLISH	GERMAN	Dosage,g
旋覆花	Xuan Fu Hua	Flos Inulae	Elecampane	Alantblüten	10
生赭石	Sheng Zhe Shi	Ochre	Ochre	Ochre	10
杏仁	Xing Ren	Semen Prumi	Apricot Seed	Aprikosensamen	10
橘红	Ju Hong	Citri Erythrocarpae	Red Tangerine	Rote Mandarinenschale	10
焦白术	Jiao Bai Zhu	Rhizoma Macrocephalae Atractylodis	Largrhead White Atractylodes (Burnt)	Großköpftig Atractylodes (Verkohltes)	10
酒黄芩	Jiu huang Qin	Scutellariae	Scute in Wine	Baikal-Helm in Wein	10

114

当归	Dang Gui	Angelicae Sinensis	Tangkuei Root	Chi. Angelikawurzel	10
白芍	Bai Shao	Paeoniae	White peony	Weiβ pfingstrosen	15
香附	Xiang Fu	Cyperi Rotundi	Cyperus Rhizoma	Nusswurzelstock	10
木瓜	Mu Gua	Chneaomelis	Chi. Quince Fruit	Chi. Quittenfrücht	10
砂仁	Sha Ren	Fructus seu Semen	Grains-of-Paradise Fruit	Amomum-Sharen-Frücht	6
藿香	Huo Xiang	Herba Agastaches	Agastache	Patchoulikraut	10

King Herb: Xuan Fu Hua, Flos Inulae (Fig. 37)

Flora: Chrysanthemum Family, Perennial, Herbaceous

Character: Bitter, Pungent, salty, warm

Meridian: Lungs, Spleen, Stomach, Large Intestine

Function: Clearing phlegm, descending adverse Qi

Component: Flavonoids, inulobiose.

Pharmacology: Xuan Fu Hua can cure nausea and vomiting owing to cold and weak of stomach and spleen. It can also cure asthma and phlegm more.

115

KING HERB	PIN YIN	旋复花 XUAN FU HUA
	LATIN	Flos Inulae
君 药	ENGLISH	Inula Flower
	GERMAN	Blüten-köpfchen von Inula

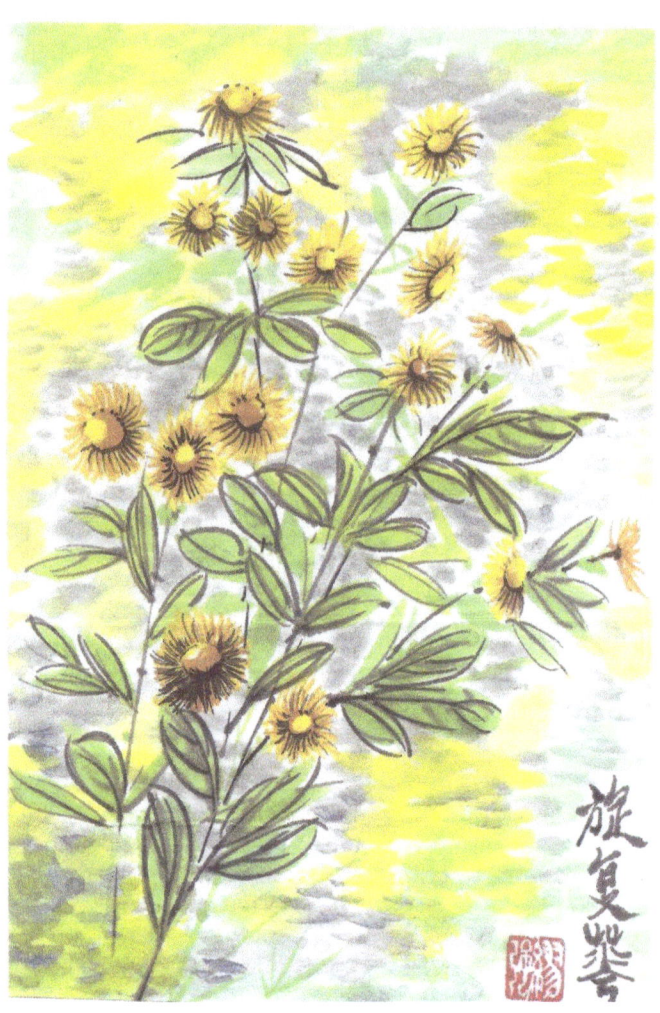

Fig. 37 Xuan Fu Hua

C. Yin weakness of liver and kidney

Syndromes: dizzy, tinnitus, deaf, pain in loins and back, sleep loss, more dreams, palpitation, irritable, easy to anger, hemorrhage of nose and teeth.

Diagnose: no tongue coating or less with white and shallow yellow colour, tongue texture: red. Pulse: thready, faint and some rapid.

Differentiation: Evil of moisture and heat blocked for long time, consumed body Qi and fluid, and then Yin of liver and kidney is weak.

Cure principle: tonifying liver and kidney.

The recipe of herbs

中文	PIN YIN	LATIN	ENGLISH	GERMANY	Dosage,g
北沙参	Bei Sha Shen	Radix Glehniae Littoralis	Northern Sand Root	Becherglocken-wurzel	30
麦门冬	Mai Men Dong	Tuber Ophiopogonis	Greeping Lily-turf Tuber	Schlangenbark-knotten	10
当归	Dang Gui	Angelicae	Tangkuei Root	Chi.Angelikawurzel	10
生地黄	Sheng Di Huang	Rehmanniae	Fresh Chinese Foxglove Root	Frische Rehmanniawurzel	10
白芍	Bai Shao	Paeoniae Lactiflorae	White Peony Root	Weiepfingstrosenwurzel	15

枸杞子	Gou Qi Zi	Fructus Lycii	Wolfberry Fruit	Bocksdorn Frücht	10
川棟子	Chuan Lian Zi	Meliae Toosendan	Sichuan Chinaberry	Paternoster-Baum-Frücht	10
木瓜	Mu Gua	Fructus Chnenomelis	Chi.Quince Fruit	Chi.Quittenfrücht	10
何首乌	He Shou Wu	Polygoni Multiflori	Fleeceflower Root	Vielblütige Knöterichwurzel	10
生甘草	Sheng Gan Cao	Ulalensis	Licorice Root	Ural-süßholzwurzel	6

King Herb: Bei Sha Shen, Radix Adenophorae (Fig. 38)

Flora: Carrot Family, Perennial, Herbaceous

Character: Sweet, Some Cold

Meridian: Lungs, Stomach, Kidney

Function: Nutrition of lungs, tonifying stomach, generating fluid

Component: Psoralen, alkaloid

Pharmacology: Antipyretic and analgesia. Stimulation of secrete of the gastric juice.

KING HERB	PIN YIN	北沙参 BEI SHA SHEN
	LATIN	Radix Glehniae Littoralis
君　药	ENGLISH	Northern Sand Root
	GERMAN	Becherglockenwurzel

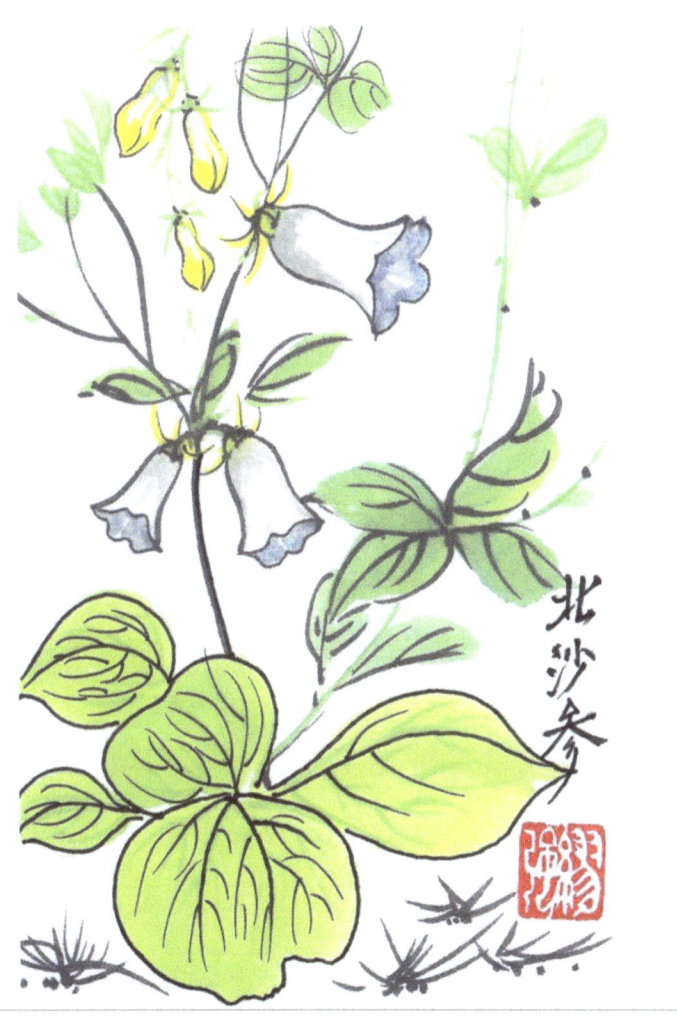

Fig. 38 Bei Sha Shen

E. Weakness of Body Qi and Blocking of Blood

Syndromes: Pain in Chest and location of pain points is obviously, liver and spleen swell; swollen lumps are hard, anorexia, acratia and breathe weakly: dysmenorrhea and with blood lumps for women.

Diagnose: face and lip: black colour. Tongue texture: withered and with spots. Pulse: thready.

Differentiation: The evil Qi of heat damages Yin of body, and consumes Yin fluid. The evil Qi of moisture damages Yang, consumes body Qi. After long time illness liver, kidney and spleen have been injured, then Qi and blood all are weak, which induces blood blocked and stasis, and the abdominal mass is formed.

Cure Principle: tonifying Qi and invigorating spleen, activating blood, to catharsis liver and conduct Qi, softening hardness and dissipating mass.

The recipe of herbs

中文	PIN YIN	LATIN	ENGLISH	GERMAN	Dosage,g
党参	Dang Shen	Radix Codonopsitis	Asiabell Root	Glockenwindenwurzel	10
黄芪	Huang Qi	Astragali	Yellow Milk-Vetch Root	Astragaluswurzel	20
当归	Dang Gui	Angelicae	Tangkuei Root	Chi.Angelikawurzel	10
白芍	Bai Shao	Radix Paeoniae	White Peony Root	Weißepfingstrosenwurzel	15
赤勺	Chi Shao	Paeoniae Rabrae	Red Peony Root	Pfingstrosenwurzel	15
丹参	Dan Shen	Salviae Miltorrhizae	Red Sage Root	Salvia-Wurzel	15

泽兰	Ze Lan	Lycopi Lucidi	Bugleweed	Wolfstrapp Kraut	15
生牡蛎	Sheng Mu Li	Ostreae	Oyster Shell	Austernschale	30
灸鳖甲	Jiu Bie Jia	Carapax Amydae	Chi. Soft-shell	Panzer der China Weichschildkröte	15
鸡内金	Ji Nei Jin	Gigeriae Galli	Chicken Gizard Lining	Hühnermagenendothel	10
藕节	Ou Jie	Nodus Neluminis	Lotus Rhizoma	Lotusrhizoma Knoten	10
香附	Xiang Fu	Cyperi Rotundi	Cyperus Rhizoma	Nusswurzelstock	10
水红花子	Shui Hong Hua Zi	Semen Carthami Tincctorii	Safflower Seed	Saflorblüten Samen	10

King Herb: Dang Shen, Radix Codonopsis (Fig. 39)

Flora: Baloonflower Family, Perennial, Herbaceous

Character: Sweet, Balance

Meridian: Spleen, Lunge

Function: Tonifying Organs, Reinforcing Qi

Component: Gledinin, alkaloid, vitamine B1, B2, inulobiose.

Pharmacology: Function of excitation for neven system, enhancement of resistance of body. Increasing content of haemoglobin and erythrocyte in blood. Dilating blood vessels and decreasing blood pressure. Inhibiting the function of high pressure of blood by adrenalin.

E. Stasis of turbid phlegm

121

Syndromes: Painful and swollen of liver and spleen, poor appetite, digest weak, dizzy, palpitation, limbs and body heavy, sleeploss or lethargy.

Diagnose: tongue texture: dark with ecchymosis, tongue is plump and with teeth-printed. Tongue coating: greasy. Pulse: slippery pulse.

Differentiation: over eating and drinking, evil Qi of moisture and heat delayed for long time in the body and the phlegm produced. Phlegm jointed with stasis blood, the liver, kidney and spleen are damaged. The fat is piled up into liver (fatty liver).

Cure principle: activating blood and resolving phlegm.

The recipe of herbs

中文	PIN YIN	LATIN	ENGLISH	GERMAN	Dosage,g
旋覆花	Xuan Fu Hua	Flos Inulae	Elecampaane	Alantblüte	10
生赭石	Sheng Zhe Shi	Ochre	Ochre	Ochre	10
橘红	Ju Hong	Citri Erythrocarpae	Red Tangerine Peel	Rote Mandarinenschale	10
赤勺	Chi Shao	Paeoniae Rubrae	Red Peony Root	Pfingstrosenwurzel	10
白芍	Bai Shao	Paeoniae	White Peony	Weißepfingstrosewurzel	10
丹参	Dan Shen	Radix Salviae	Red Soge Root	Salvia-Wurzel	10
香附	Xiang Fu	Cyperi	Cyperus rhizoma	Nusswurzelstock	10

瓜蒌	Gua Lou	Trichosanthis	Snakegourd	Schlangenkürbis	15
小蓟	Xiao Ji	Cephalanoplos	Small Thistle	Cephalanoplos	10
藕节	Ou Jie	Nodus Nelumbinis	Lotus Rhizoma Node	Lutosrhizomknoten	10
泽兰	Ze Lan	Lycopi Lucidi	Bugleweed	Wolfstrappkraut	10

King herb: Xuan Fu Hua.

**Above 5 pieces of recipes are from Prof. Guan, You Bo. Beijing, China. The analysis of syndroms is from Prof. Zhao, Bo Zhi 《The Explanation of Hepatothies Cases by Guan, You Bo, Nov. 2007》

KING HERB	PIN YIN	党参 DANG SHEN
	LATIN	Radix Codonopsis
君 药	ENGLISH	Pilose Asiabell Root
	GERMAN	Glockenwindenwurzel

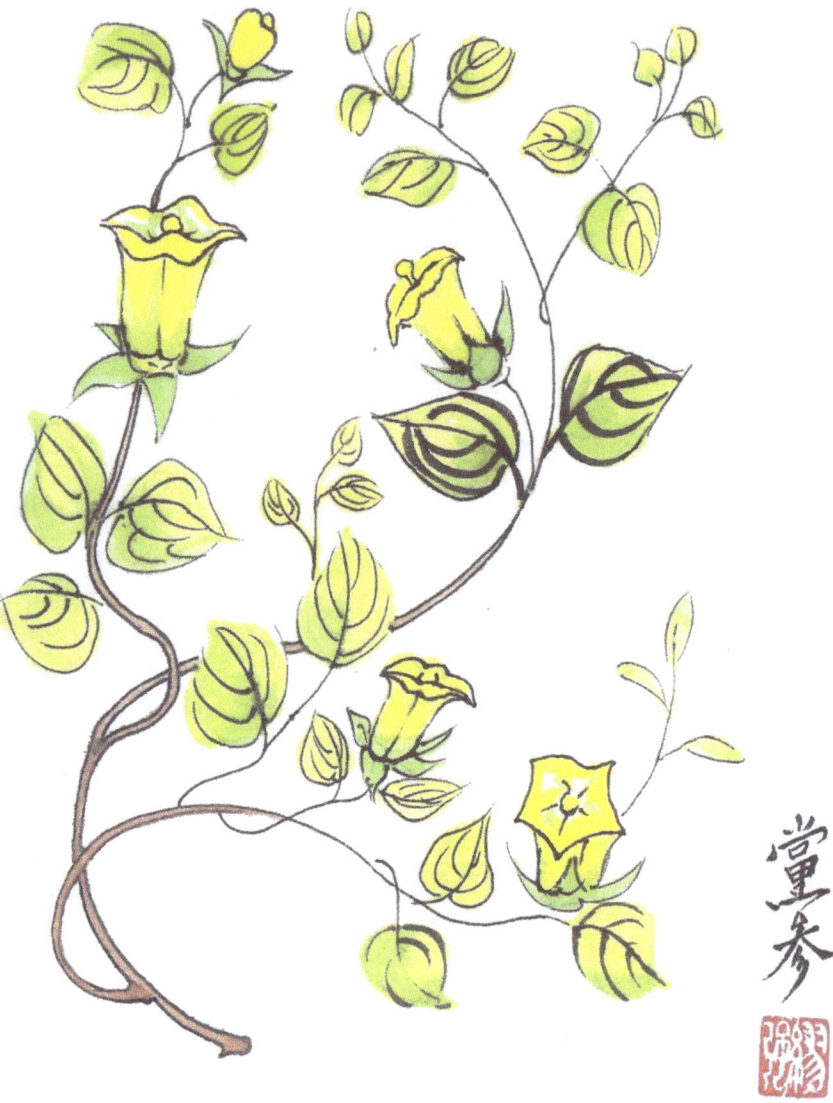

Fig. 39 Dang Shen

7.3.2. Case

Case 1

Name: Mr. Li, M, 25, used to be a patient of acute icterohepatitis. 17, Aug. 1993 first visiting.

Syndromes: Icterus happened again, tired and acratia, abdominal distension, stool watery and mashed.

Diagnose of West Medicine: Chronic hepatitis B.

Illness-Name of TCM: Yang Huang.

Diagnose of Chinese Medicine: Icterus happened again means spleen weakness, Qi and blood not enough. Evil Qi of moisture blocks Zhong Jiao (Middle Energizer), Spleen losses digesting function, evil Qi of moisture injured organs again, and then icterus appears once more.

Cure principle: reinforcing spleen, regulating and tonifying Qi and blood of body, at same time catharsising liver and blood.

The herbs of Dang Shen, Fu Ling, Zhu Ling and Gan Cao (Four Gentlemen Decoction) are for tonifying spleen and stomach. Herbs of Dang Gui, Bai Shao, Chi Shao and Dan Shen are for tonifying and regulating blood. Jiao San Xian, Zhi Qiao reinforcing stomach, regulating Qi and resolving abdominal distension. The else herbs are for clearing moisture and heat, resolving toxic, clearing and cooling blood.

The recipe of herbs

中文	PIN YIN	LATIN	ENGLISH	GERMAN	Dosage,g
党参	Dang Shen	Miltiorrhizae	Red Sage Root	Salvia-Wurzel	15
白术	Bai Zhu	Rhizoma Macrocephalae Atractylodis	Largrhead White Atractylodes	Groβköpftig Atractylodes	15
猪苓	Zhu Ling	Polypori	Polyporus	Porling	30
生甘草	Sheng Gan Cao	Radix Glycyrrhizae	Liquorice Root	Ural-Süholz-Wurzel	6
当归	Dang Gui	Angelicae	Tangkuei	Chi. Angelika	12
丹参	Dan Shen	Radix Salviae	Red Sage Root	Salvia-Wurzel	12
赤勺	Chi Shao	Paeoniae Rubrae	Red Peony Root	Pfingstrose	12
白芍	Bao Shao	Paeoniae	White Peony	Weiβepfingstrose	12
蚤休	Zao Xiu	Rhizoma Paradis	Paris Rhizoma	Einbewenwurzel	10
刘寄奴	Liu Ji Nu	Herb Artemisiae	Artemisia	Schwefel	12
水红花子	Shui Hong Hua Zi	Carthami Tinctorii	Sufflower Seed	Saflorblütensamen	18
土茯苓	Tu Fu Ling	Rhizoma Smilacis	Glabrous Greenbrier	Stechwindenwurzel	30
郁金	Yu Jin	Tuber Curcumae	Tumeric Tuber	Gelbwurzknolle	10
虎杖	Hu Zhang	Polygoni Cuspidati	Giant Knotweed	Reynoutria-Wurzel stock	10
焦三鲜	Jiao San Xian		Burnt Bread	Verkohlter Brot	15
枳壳	Zhi Qiao	Fructus Anrantii	Orange Fruit	Orange	10

126

King Herb: Dang Shen, Radix Codonopsis (Fig. 39)

After drinking 10 doses of Decoctions, GOT became normally, Antigen of Hepatitis B: Negative. The symptoms of fatigue, non-appetite and abdominal distension all are disappeared. After drinking 15 doses of this decoctions again, the patient recovered healthy and continued to work.

**This recipe is from Prof. Wu, Jun Yu, Beijing, China.

Minister Herb: Bai Zhu, Rhizom Atractylodis Macrocephalae (Fig. 40)

Flora: Composite Family, Perennial, Herbacerous

Character: Bitter, sweet, warm

Meridian: Spleen, Stomach

Function: Tonifying spleen, clearing moisture and water, relieving sweat

Component: Volatile (atractylol, atractylone), vitamin A

Pharmacology: Protection of liver to prevent reduction of glycogen. Conducting of urine, promoting of excretion of electrolytes. Volatile has the function of analgesia and decreasing blood glucose.

MINISTER HERB	PIN YIN	白术 BAI ZHU
	LATIN	Rhizoma Atractylodis Macrocephalae
臣 药	ENGLISH	Largehead Atractylodes Rhizome
	GERMAN	Großköpfige Atractylodeswurzel

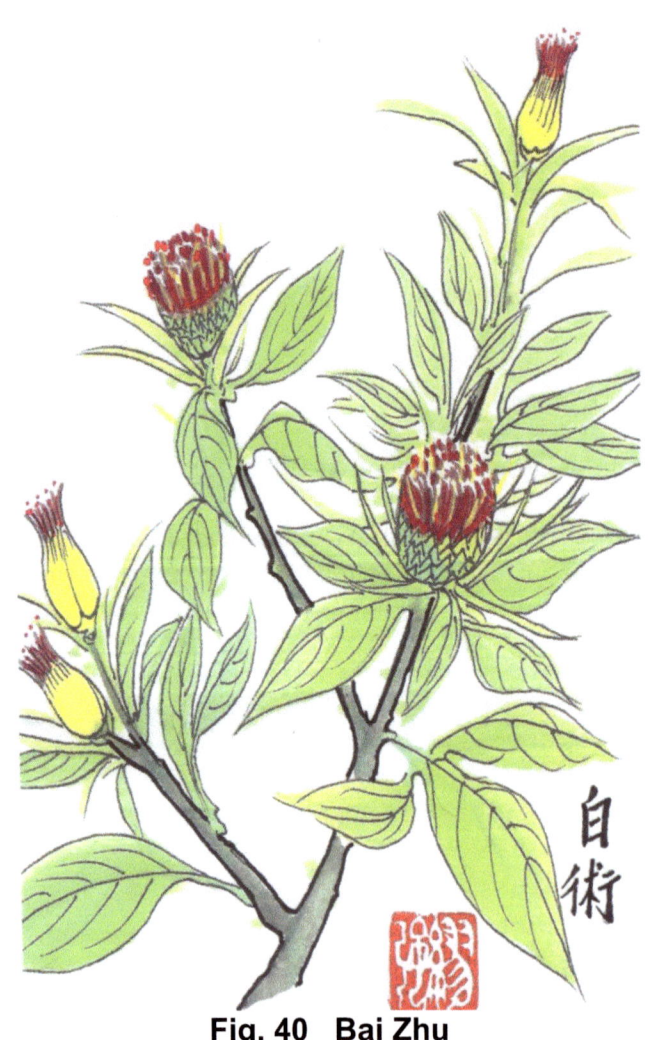

Fig. 40   Bai Zhu

128

Name: Mr. Sun, M. 43, 18, May 1989 first visiting.

From 1986 the patient always pained in chest, and was acratic, fatigue, urine is yellow. Diagnosis was confirmed of chronic hepatitis. In recent three months, due to disturb of emotion the illness situation became seriously and icterus appeared.

Laboratory datum: GPT 130, icteric index 18, TTT 11, urine bilirubin, urobilin and urobilinogen: Positive.

Diagnosis of West Medicine: Chronic Hepatitis.

Diagnose of TCM: Shallow red of tongue texture, white and greasy coating. Pulse: deep, wiry and weak.

Illness Name of TCM: Yin Huang.

Differentiation: Middle Yang (digest) is weak, spleen and stomach are deficiency, Qi of cold and moisture blocked, "declining of liver produces innerior cold" <Tai Ping Sheng Hui Fang 太平圣惠方>，cold resists the function of catharsis of liver, Qi mechanism is blocked.

Cure principle: reinforcing spleen and regulating Middle Yang, the innerior cold evil can be resolved by warm herbs, reinforcing Middle Yang, activating blood and resolving stasis.

The recipe of herbs

中文	PIN YIN	LATIN	ENGLISH	GERMAN	Dosage,g
生黄芪	Sheng Huang Qi	Astragali	Yellow-Milk -Vetch	Astragaluswurzel	30
嫩桂枝	Nen Gui Zhi	Cinnamomi Cassiae	Fresh Cinnamon Twig	Frische Zimtzweige	6
炒白芍	Chao Bai Shao	Paeoniae	Fried White Peony Root	Gebratene Weiße Pfingstrosewurzel	30
土扁豆	Tu Bian Dou	Semen Dolichoris Lablab	Hyacinth Bean	Helmbohnensamen	15
白茯苓	Bai Fu Ling	Poriae Cocos	White Hoelen	Weiße Kokospilz	30
金钱草	Jin Qian Cao	Herb Lysimachiae	Christina Loosestrife	Felberich	9
炙甘草	Jiu Gan Cao	Radix Glycyrrhizae	Toast Liquorice Root	Rösten Ural-Süßholz-Wurzel	9
生姜	Sheng Jiang	Rhizoma Zingiberis	Fresh Ginger	Frische Ingwerwurzel	9
大枣	Da Zao	Ziziphi Jujubbee	Chi. Black Date	Dattelfrucht	3 pie.
六神曲	Liu Shen Qu	Liu Shen Qu	Liu Shen Qu	Liu Shen Qu	3
第 2 方加			Second Recipe plus		
呼延索	Hu Yan Suo	Corydalis	Corydalis	Lerchensporenwurzelstock	15
牡丹皮	Mu Dan Pi	Cotex Muutan Radicis	Tree Peony Rootbark	Strauchpaeonien Wurzelrinde	9
白茅根	Bai Mao Gen	Rhizoma Cylindricae	White Grass Rhizome	Alang-Alang-Gras Wurzelstock	30
车前草	Che Qian Cao	Herba Plantaginis	Plantago	Wegerich	5

King Herbs: Huang Qi (Fig. 36)

After drinking 9 doses of this decoction, the Lab. Test: icteruse index 5, TTT 9, GPT 80, urine bilirubin, urobilin and urobilinogen all are negative. According this receipt, 7 doses drinking again, and all index are normally. Following up half year, the illness has not relapsed.

**This case and recipe is from Prof. Qiao, Bao Jun, Luoyang, China.

Minister Herb: Gui Zhi, Cassia Twig (Fig. 41)

Flora: Camphor Family, Evergreen Arbor, small leaves

Character: Pungent, sweet, warm

Meridian: Heart, Lungs, Bladder

Function: Conducting Yang, eliminating cold, clearing moisture

In this recipe, Huang Qi is tonifying body Qi, Gui Zhi and Bian Dou are warming the body's Yang, dispelling moisture, reinforcing catharsis. Bai Shao is activating blood.

Component: volatile (cinnamaldehyde, cinnamate)

Pharmacology: Stimulation of secrete of sweat gland, dilatation of vessels of skin, antipyretic analgesic. Promoting secrete of saliva and gastric juice. Relieving spasm of smooth muscle of organs, remove abdominal pain. Dilatating artery of heart muscle with function of cardiotonic.

MINISTER HERB 臣 药	PIN YIN	桂枝 GUI ZHI
	LATIN	Ramulus Cinnamomi Cassiae
	ENGLISH	Cassia Twig
	GERMAN	Zimtzweig oder Cassiazweige

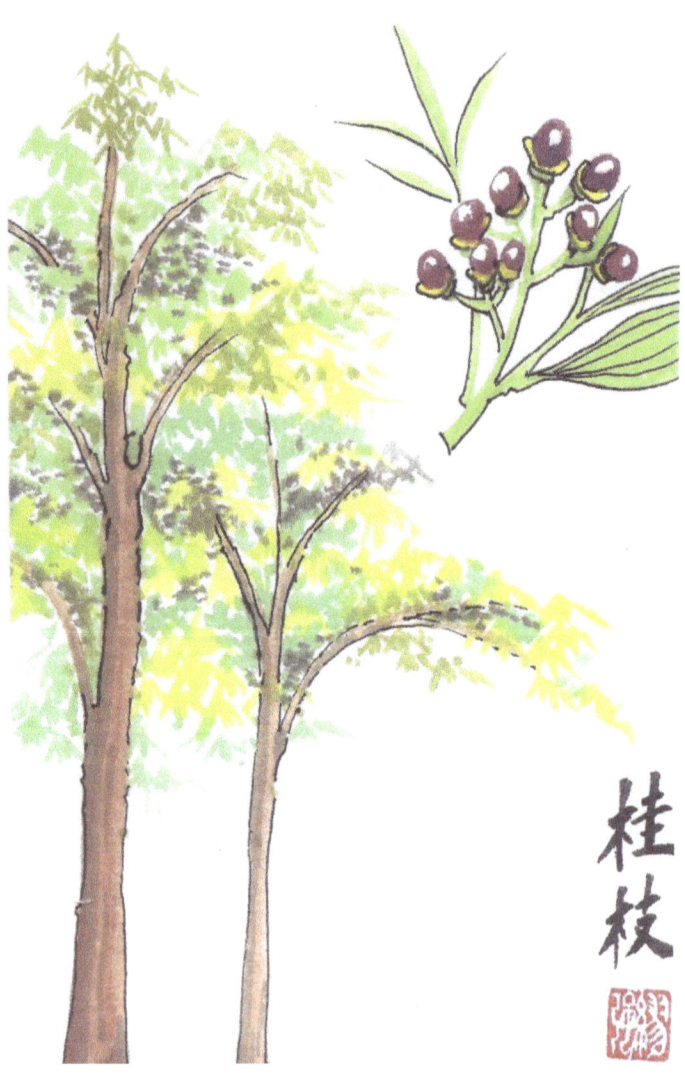

桂枝

Fig. 41 Gui Zhi

7.4. Hepatocirrhose

Generally speaking Hepatocirrhose is developed from chronic hepatitis. Its name in TCM is "Ji Ju（积聚）". The persistent time is from several months to several ten years. It's possible to change into hepatocirrhose from all the types of hepatitis A, B, C, D and E, the changing probability is about one third. The hepatocirrhoses are divided to two kinds of earlier state (compensatory phase) and lateral state (non-compensatory phase). The lateral phase of hepatotitis is always acompanied with ascites.

7.4.1. Cause and Mechanism of Illness

The cause of hepatocirrhose is owing to the cure in the period of chronic hepatitis is unsuitable or not thorough, and chronic hepatitis repeatedly breaks out. The evils of moisture and heat detained interior, and puzzle spleen and liver. Qi and blood are lost and debility, and Yin fluid is not enough, phlegm and moisture joint together and the abdominal mass produces.

The blood circulation is obstructed which induces varicosis of abdominal wall and esophagus, Further the spleen losses the fuction of controlling blood, hemorrhage of nose and esophagus is seriously happened.

If patients have the custom of excessive drinking of alcohol, and work overload, or have been stimulated strongly by emotion and can't be free themselves, it's easy to change into hepatocirrhose from chronic hepatitis.

7.4.2. The Principle of Therapy by TCM

Hepatocirrhose is a chronic, progressive and diffusive hepatitis. The Pathology is the liver cells change characters, necrosis and regenerate diffusively, and then the hyperplasia of connective tissues is happened. The construction of hepatic lobules are damaged, pseudolobulis are formed which makes liver harder gradually. Due to there are not the virucidal drugs and the

virus always hide into the liver's cells, the invasion is always happened, so the therapy is very difficult.

On the other hand, the therapy by TCM is based on the principle of "Qi" and "Xue (Blood)". In the condition of co-existence of human body and mass, the Qi and Xue (especially Qi) could be regulated with herbs, acupuncture or qigong exercises which can produce the follows effects: enhance the action of bio-wave to the membrane of liver cells, regulate the movement and fluidity of membrane, promote blood micro-circulation, increase the function of metabolism and exchange of substances and energy, improve the immunity to phagocytize virus more, stop the transform of liver cells to connective tissues, transfomer the injured cells into normal cells, at same time enlarge division and renewing of the normal cells to replace dead cells, realize the recovery of liver capability gradually.

7.4.3. Differentiation and Cure

There are three situations for the differentiation of the syndromes of hepatocirrhose.

A. Yang weakness of spleen, liver and kidney; Qi weakened and Blood blocked

Due to long time of chronic hepatitis the dysfunction of spleen in digestion appears, and then the Kidney Yang is deficient. On the other side the digestion of spleen and stomach all need the warming and nutrition by kidney, so at least the Yang of spleen, liver and kidney totally become weak and degenerated. The result is Qi and Blood are blocked and stasis is produced.

In curing at first the Qi of liver and spleen must be reinforced, at same time warming the Yang of kidney and spleen, as well as activating blood and resolving stasis are necessary.

Case

Name: Liu, W. 54, chronic hepatitis 2 years, the situation becomes incuriously serious with pain in chest, anoresia, less urine, abdominal distension, absentminded, legs swollen lightly.

Laboratory Test: TTT 11, GPT 56, albumin 23 g/L, globulin 28.8 g/L, icteric index 9, ultra-sonic: numerous minute echoes, and sight of septates echoes, possibility of ascite.

Diagnosis by West medicine: Earlier Hepatocirrhose.

Diagnosis by Chinese medicine: tongue texture: violet colour, coating: greasy with white colour. Pulse: deep, wiry and thready.

Illness name by TCM: Ji Jü, Zheng (积聚，癥).

Differentiation: perplexed by moisture and heat long time, Qi and Blood blocked, spleen and liver damaged, kidney Yang is weak,

Cure Principle: warmly tonifying spleen and kidney, reinforcing Qi and resolving stasis.

The recipe of herbs：

中文	PIN YIN	LATIN	ENGLISH	GERMAN	Dosage,g
黄芪	Huang Qi	Astragali	Yellow Milk-Vetch	Astragaluswurzel	30
当归	Dang Gui	Angelicae	Tangkuei	Chi. Angelika	10
茯苓	Fu Ling	Poriae Cocos	Hoelen	Kokospilz	12
干姜	Gan Jiang	RhizomaZingiberis	Dried Ginger	Getrocknete Ingwer	2
白术	Bai Zhu	Rhizoma Macrocephalae Atractylodis	Largrhead White Atractylodes	Großköpftig Atractylodes	10

135

熟地黄	Shu Di Huang	Radix Rehmanniae Glutinosae Conquitae	Wine-cooked Chinese Foxglove Root	Rehmanniawurzel in Wein gekocht	15
益母草	Yi Mu Cao	Herba Leonuri Heterophylli	Motherwort	Chi. Muterkraut	100
泽兰叶	Ze Lan Ye	Lycopi Lucidi	Bugeleweed	Wolfstrappwurzel	30
甘草	Gan Cao	Rhizoma Glycyrrhizae	Liquorice Root	Ural- Sü β holz-Wurzel	10

The King Herb of this receipt is Huang Qi. (Fig. 36)

In this recipe the function of Huang Qi is ascending and tonifying spleen. Dang Gui and Gan Jiang can warm and reinforces Yang of spleen and kidney. Bai Zhu invigorates spleen, Shu Di Huang notifies kidney, big amount of Yi Mu Cao and Ze Lan can activate blood and resolve stasis. Continue to drink 5 doses of above recipe, appetite and sleeping of patient is better, urine fluently, abdominal distension and swollen free.

In next two months, the two herbs of Yi Mu Cao and Ze Lang removed out and plus Huai Shan Yao, the patient took the new recipe for two months, the albumin: globulin is changed to 38.8g/30.0g. After half year patient was fully recovered.

**These recipes and case are from Prof. Zhu, Liang Chun, Nantong, China.

The Minister Herb is Dang Gui, Root of Chinese Angelica (Fig. 42)

Flora: Perennial herbaceous carrot family.

Character: Sweat, pungent, warm.

Meridian: liver, heart, spleen.

Function: Tonic for blood, activating blood, analgesic.

Component: Volatile (monoterpenoids and sesquiterpennoids), Water soluble alkaloid, succinic acid, pellagramin, β -sitosterol, vitamine E, B12.

Pharmrcology: Protection for liver and kidney, especially the glycogen of liver. Increasing circulation and hematopoiesis function.

MINISTER HERB	PIN YIN	当归 DANG GUI
	LATIN	Radix Angelicae Sinensis
臣 药	ENGLISH	Chinese Angelica Root
	GERMAN	Chinesische Engelwurz

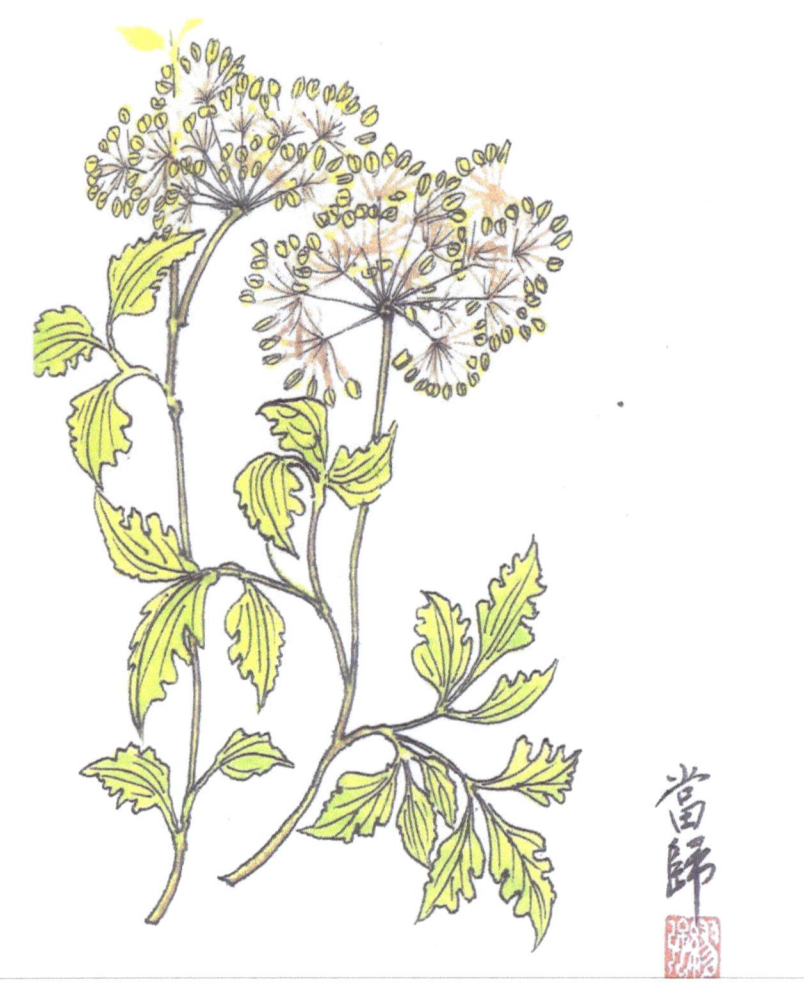

Fig. 42   Dang Gui

B. Yin weakness of liver and kidney, deficiency of Qi and stasis of blood

As a result of the evil Qi of heat and moisture stayed in blood for a long time, the Yin fluid of liver and kidney were much more consumed, and Yin weakness of liver and kidney has appeared. Yin weakness produces interior Fire, this fire joints with evil Qi of heat and moisture, and the stasis and hepatocirrhose would appear.

Case:

Name: Mr. Zhou, 28. from 1961 the patient felt acratia, with light swollen. 1962 the function of liver was not normal. In Feb. 1963 first visiting to us. Face is with black-grey colour, there were Vascular spider in face and hand, liver can be toughed subcostal, the spleen was bigger 1cm and pain. Needle biopsy of liver: nodular cirrhosis. Contrast: varicosis of esophagus.

Diagnosis by West Medicine: Hepatocirrhosis.

Diagnosis by Chinese Meidcine: Tongue texture: red colour, Coating: white colour, Pulse: deep, thready, slippery.

Name of TCM: Ji Jü. Jia (积聚，瘕)

Differentiation: Impairment of Yin essence of liver and kidney, dysfunction of spleen in digestion and transportation, weakness of body's Qi and blood blocked, meridian resisted by stasis and blood.

Cure principle: tonifying liver and kidney, invigorating spleen and reinforcing Qi, nutrition for liver-blood, nourishing liver, activating blood and conducting meridian.

The recipe of herbs

中文	PIN YIN	LATIN	ENGLISH	GERMAN	Dosage,g
生黄芪	Huang Qi	Astragali	Yellow-Milk-Vetch	Astragaluswurzel	15
白芍	Bai Shao	Paeoniae	White Peony	Weiß epfingstrose	30
女贞子	Nü Zhen Zi	Fructus Ligustri Lucidi	Waxtree Fruit	Ligusterfrücht	15
党参	Dang Shen	Radix Codonopsitis	Asiabell Root	Glockenwindenwurzel	12
菟丝子	Tu Si Zi	Semen Cuscutae Chinensis	Dodder Seed	Chi. Teufelszwimsamen	15
川续断	Xü Duan	Radix Dipsaci Asperi	Teasel Root	Chin. Kardenwurzel	25
木瓜	Mu Gua	Frucht Chaenomelis	Chi. Quince Fruit	Chi. Quittenfrüchte	12
阿胶珠	E Jiao	Corii Asini	Ass Skin Glue	Eselshaut-Gelatine	9
白术	Bai Zhu	Rhizoma Macrocephalae Atractylodis	Largrhead White Atractylodes	Großköpftig Atractylodes	9
地榆	Di Yü	Radix Sanguisorbae	Bumet-Blood wort Root	Wiesenknopfwurzel	15
茵陈	Yin Chen	Artemisiae Scopariae	Virgate Wormwood	Besenbeifußkraut	15
藿香	Huo Xiang	Herb Pogostemonis	Cablin Patchoulikraut	Patchoulikraut	6
蒲公英	Po Gong Ying	Herb Taraxaci	Dandelion	Löwenzahnkraut	15
小蓟	Xiao Ji	Cephalanoplos	Small Thistle	Cephalanoplos	15
乌梅炭	Wu Mei Tan	Frutus Pruni Mume	Burnt Ume Plum Fruit	Verkohlter Umeaprikosenfrüchte	3

140

Patient drank this recipe for 4 months. From Jun. 1963 the recipe was changed to follows:

中文	PIN YIN	LATIN	ENGLISH	GERMAN	Dosage,g
黄芪	Huang Qi	Astragali	Yellow Milk-Vetch	Astragaluswurzel	30
当归	Dang Gui	Angelicae	Tangkuei	Chi. Angelika	12
地黄	Di Huang	Rhizoma Rehmanniae	Chi. Foxglove Root	Rehmanniawurzel	15
何首乌	He Shou Wu	Radix Polygoni Multiflori	Fleeceflower Root	Vielblütig Knöterichwurzel	30
白芍	Bai Shao	Paeoniae	White Peony	Weißepfingstrose	30
青蒿	Qing Hao	Artemisiae Aunuae	Sweet Wormwood	Einjähriges Beifuβ kraut	12
黄连	Huang Lian	Coptidis	Coptis	Goldfadenwurzel	6
败酱草	Bai Jiang Cao	Potriniae	Potrinia	Patrinia	9
延胡索	Yan Hu Suo	Corydalis	Corydalis	Lerchensporen Wurzelstock	9
木瓜	Mu Gua	Frucht Chaenomelis	Chi. Quince Fruit	Chi. Quittenfrüchte	12
茵陈	Yin Chen	Artemisiae Scopariae	Virgate Wormwood	Besenbeif kraut	15
乌梅	Wu Mei	Fructus Prumi Mume	Ume Plum Fruit	Umeaprikosenfrücht	9
地榆	Di Yü	Radix Sanguisorbae	Bumet-Blood wort Root	Wiesenknopfwurzel	15
小蓟	Xiao Ji	Cephalanoplos	Small Thistle	Cephalanoplos	15
甘草	Gan Cao	Radix Glycyrrhizae	Liquorice Root	Ural-Süßholz-Wurzel	3

This recipe was taken to the end of 1965. In 1966 interrupted drinking. In the test in May 1970, varicosis was not seen in the contrast of esophagus, patient recovered healthy.

**This case and recipe are from Prof. Guan, You Bo, Beijing, China.

Here must be emphasised that in these recipes there are only tonifying herbs for activating Qi and blood, conducting meridian, and reinforcing essence and nourishing Yin. But the doctor did not use the attacking, expelling and purgative herbs, such as Da Ji (Radix Knoxiae), Gan Sui (Radix Kansui), Da Huang (Fibraureae Recisa), Bai Hua She She Cao (Rubiaceae) , etc. Otherwise the serious situation would be happened such as esophagus vein broken.

C. Yin deficiency with heat blood, Qi deficiency and blood stasis

The syndromes are as follows: hemorrhage of mouth or nose, vexing heat in chest, palms and soles, dry of stool, urine short and with red colour, rosy cheek, night sweat, vascular spider in palms and face. Some of patients have poisoning history of pharmacy or foods. Liver was damaged seriously and then bigger and harder.

Case

Name: Wang, M. 46. In Jul. 1971 due to light fever the patient was misdiagnosed as malaria, took big amount of quinine, and then liver damaged.

Laboratory datum: (Dec. 1971) bilirubin, urobilin and urobilinogen all are positive, ALT: 495U /L, TTT: 29, haemoglobin 10g /L, leukocyte 5200 /L, platelet 9400 /L, blood sedimentation 69 mm/h, icterus index 12, alkaline phosphatase 5U, albulin / globulin: 2.6 / 4.4. There were a 6cm mass in subcoastal liver, and a mass 8cm in subxiphoid, all were smooth.

The first visiting to us is in March 1973, ALT 520U/L, TTT 20. Black face, vexing emotion, much more dreams, hemorrhage from nose and teeth, cinnabar palms.

Diagnosis by West Medicine: Earlier Hepatocirrhose

Diagnosis by TCM: tongue texture: red colour, coating: white, pulse: wiry

III Name of TCM: Ji Jü, Zheng (积聚，癥)

Cure principle: tonifying Qi and reinforcing Yin, cooling and activating blood.

The recipe of herbs

中文	PIN YIN	LATIN	ENGLISH	GERMAN	Dosage,g
黄芪	Huang Qi	Astragali	Yellow Milk-Vetch	Astragaluswurzel	24
地黄	Di Huang	Rhizoma Rehmanniae	Chi. Foxglove Root	Rehmanniawurzel	15
白芍	Bai Shao	Paeoniae	White Peony	Weißepfingstrose	15
丹参	Dan Shen	Miltiorrhizae	Red Sage Root	Salvia-Wurzel	24
藕节	Ou Jie	Nodus Nelumbinis	Lotus Rhizoma Node	Lotusrhizomknoten	12
红花	Hong Hua	Flos Carthami Tinctorii	Safflower	Saflorblüte	15
泽兰	Ze Lan	Herb Lycopi	Bugleweed	Wolfstrappkraut	15
草河车	Cao He Che	Rhizoma Paridis	Paris Rhizome	Einbewenwurzel	15

木瓜	MU Gua	Frucht Chaenomulis	Chi. Quince Fruit	Chi. Quittenfrüchte	12
阿胶	E Jiao	Corii Asini	Ass Skin Glue	Eselshaut-Gelatine	9
郁金	Yü Jin	Tuber Curcumae	Tumeric Tuber	Gelbwurzelknolle	12
王不留行	Wang Bu Liu Xing	Semen Vaccariae Segetalis	Cow Soapwort Seed	Kuhkrautsamen	12
槐花炭	Huai Hua Tan	Flos Sophorae	Burnt Pagoda Tree Flower	Verkohte Schnurbaum blüte	12

In this recipe there is a big amount of Huang Qi which could tonify body Qi effectly, Bai Shao, Dan Shen and E Jiao can reinforce blood and soften stasis of liver, Cao He Che, Di Huang, Ou Jie and Huai Hua can remove out heat, detoxicate, cool blood and stanch bleeding. Hong Hua, Ze Lan, Wang Bu Liu Xing can activate blood and dissipate stasis. Yü Jin, Mu Gua can catharsis liver and regulate Qi.

After drinking of 14 doses of above receipt, the function of liver has been better. ALT 142 U/L, TTT 6.5U. And also took this receipt for half year. Recheck in April 1974: albumin / globumin: 4.6 / 3.2, the fuction of liver all are normally.

**This case and recipe are from Prof. Guan, You Bo, Beijing, China.

7.5. Ascites due to Cirrhose

Ascites is the lateral period of decompensatory cirrhose. Its name in TCM is "Shui Gu" (水臌, water swollen), or "石水" (Shi Shui, stone water). Before 2500 years 《灵枢 Ling Shu●水胀篇 Shui Zhang Pian》 has pointed out: "Shui Gu is abdominal distension, body and limbs all become thicker and same as abdominal swollen, skin is with sallow colour, the vessels on abdomen bulge. The above symptoms are the syndrome of Shui Gu".

7.5.1. The Disease Causes and Mechanism

《Su Wen 素问》said, "The exhaustion of Yang Qi is meaning swollen." This illustrated swollen is induced by weakness of Yang Qi (energy). Dr. Zhang, Jing Yü, famous Doctor in Ming dynasty (A.D.1368-1644) pointed out: "Swollen has relation with the organ of lungs, spleen and kidney interactively".

"Wu Xing 五行" Principles recognize, "Wood controls earth", Owing to the long period of chronic hepatitis, function of spleen and stomach is damaged, essence of after birth is not enough. Due to "Earth produces metal", the Yin of lungs is deficiented and damaged, the lungs' function of arranging water decreases. Due to "Metal produces water", the Yin of kidney is also damaged. For a long time, the Yang of kidney has been exhausted. Kidney is the gate of water, so it is unsuccessful of closing gate. The water and moisture are blocked interiorly and the swollen is formed.

7.5.2. Differentiation and Cure

The cure and differentiation of ascites of cirrhose should start from reinforcing and tonifying the Yin of spleen, lungs and kidney. Kidney is the Qi resource inborn. Tonifying spleen means vitality of earth, and earth can produce metal (lungs) and water (Kidney), when water of kidney is enough, the original Qi of the body is vigorously. Tonifying the Yin of lungs makes the function of arranging water in the body stronger. When function of lungs and kidney recover, the tunnels of water conducted, the symptome of ascites disappears automatically.

The ascites of cirrhose is the lateral period of cirrhose, the situation of illness is complicated. There are either excess pathogenic Qi of moisture and heat, or deficiency of Yin. There are either warm of blood, or body Qi's deficiency. There is the deficiency in excess; and also, there is the excess in deficiency. **But we must know that for this illness we must give priority to the deficiency of body's Qi, but to remove the excess of pathogenic evil is auxiliary only.** From the principle of "reinforcing healthy Qi and eliminating pathogenic excess", after tonifying Yin, invigorating Yang and regulating Qi and Blood, ascites will be disappeared naturally.

The methods of TCM to cure ascites of cirrhose is "seeing water but not treat water", "seeing blood but not treat blood." For ascites, especially for the serious ascites, TCM does not advocate to releasing water by intubation. Because this method is extremely possible to disrupt the balance of electrolyte and also loss much more protein. In Tang Dynasty (A.D.618-907) the great expert of TCM, Dr. Sun, Si Miao in his works of 《千金方》 (Qian Jin Fang) said, "Abstain from releasing water in abdomen, otherwise be dead within one month possibly." At same time in herb recipe it is forbidden to use attacking and aggressive herbs for catharsising and releasing water and oedema, such as E Shu (莪术 Turmeric Rhizome), San Leng (三棱 Rhizoma Sparganii), etc. which should make the illness much more serious. For hemorrhage of nose and mouth, it's better to use the method of tonifying Qi, activating Blood and resolving stasis.

The differentiation of the ascites of cirrhose may be divided three situations.

A. Damage and deficiency of kidney Yang, Blocking of water and moisture.

Due to a long time of illness of hepatocirrhosis, the Yin of spleen, lunge and kidney are damaged, at same time the Yang of kidney also be lost, and the original Qi of body becomes deficiency. The kidney controls tunnels of water, and now open and close are out of control, so the retention of water and moisture happen.

Case

Name: Chen, M. 27. Patient used to spit out big amount of blood, and with abdominal ascites. "Portal cirrhosis" was diagnosed, then spleen was abscised and the ligature of veins (left and right) of stomach was operated. Later patient was transferred to us and has the first visiting. The patient's abdomen swollen was seriously, the circumference of abdomen was 87.5cm, the veins of esophagus were totally varicosis.

Laboratory Test: albumin: 20.2g /L, globulin: 35.3g /L, TTT: 9, TFT: +++, CCFT: +++.

Diagnose of West Medicine: Severe Ascites of hepatocirrhosis.

Diagnose of TCM: Tongue texture: bright, Coating: less, Pulse: deep, thready.

Name of TCM: Shui Gu (水臌)。

Differentiation and Cure: patient has been operated two times, ascites was very heavy, the vein of esophsgus are all varicosis. The patient's situation was exacerbation, and belonged to "Yang Deficiency" from the diagnosis of tongue and pulse. 《Su Wen》 said, "the swollen owing to Qi weakness, that means Yang Qi has been exhausted totally". Spleen, liver and kidney all were deficiency. The True Essence Fire (Energy 真火) in Ming Men (Life Gate 命门, a very important Acu-point, BL23 in Bladder meridian) has been lost, the water could not be transferred and evaporated, kidney closed the tunnel and the water was gathered.

In cure treatment it is necessary to reinforce the True Yin (真阴) and True Yang（真阳）of spleen, lungs and kidney. **If the Yang is vitality, the superfluous "Yin Water (阴水)" (which has been produced from damaged organs and gathered in the distension of abdominal and limbs) can be removed out. If the Yin is vitality, the superfluous "Yang Water (阳 水)" (which is from outside, such as every day's drinking and transfusion from outside) can be also removed out normally.**

The recipe of herbs

中文	PIN YIN	LATIN	ENGLISH	GERMAN	Dosage,g
熟地黄	Shu Di Huang	Radix Rehmanniae Glutinosae Conquitae	Wine-Cooked Chi. Foxlove Root	Rehmanniawurzel in Wein gekocht	18
山萸肉	Shan Yu Rou	Fructus Cormi Officinalis	Dogwood Fruit	Kornelkirchenfrüchte	9
茯苓	Fu Ling	Poriae	Hoelen	Kokospilz	12
桂枝	Gui Zhi	Ramulus Cinnamomi Cassiae	Cinnamon Twig	Zimtzeige	4.5
山药	Shan Yao	Radix Dioscoreae Oppositae	Chi. Wild Yam Root	Yamswurzelknollen	9
牡丹皮	Mu Dan Pi	Cortex Moutan Radicis	Tree Peony Rootbark	Strauchpaeonien-Wurzelrinde	4.5
泽泻	Ze Xie	Rhizoma Alismatis Orientalitis	Water Plantain Rhizome	Orient-Froschlöffelknollen	6
八味地黄丸	Ba Wei Di Huang Wan		Set Presscription of Chinese Herbs		4.5
淡附片	Dan Fu Pian	Radix Lateralis Aconiti Carmichaeli Peaeparata	Prepared Sichuan Aconite Root	Vorbehandelte Eisenhutseitenwurzel	4.5

**This case and recipe are from Prof. Yan, De Xin, Shanghai, China

In this recipe Shu Di Huang and Shan Yu Rou tonify liver and kidney, Shan Zhu Yi tonifies spleen, Shan Yao tonifies Qi, Fu Ling and Ze Xie conduct water tunnels. All the herbs can make kidney Qi abundant, Yin and Yang balance, the ascites distension would be disappeared automatically.

After taking several doses of above recipe, the amount of urine increased day and day, average 1000 ml per day, the circumference of abdomen was decreased to 80cm. albumin: globulin is 40.8 : 35.2, TTT: 4, TFT: +/-.

The patient continuously took above recipe (for removing the else evil moisture and heat, plus 15g of Huang Qi, 9g of Niu Xi and 9g of Che Qian Zi). The total course of treatment was one year. At least the circumference abdomen was reduced to 74cm, function of liver was normal again.

**This case and recipe are from Prof. Yan, De Xin, Shanghai, China

King Herb: Shu Di Huang, Radix Rehmannie Praepareta (Fig. 43)

Flora: Scrophulariaceae, Perennial, Herbaceous.

Character: sweet, warm.

Meridian: Heart, Liver, Kidney.

Effect: Tonifying heart, reinforcing Yin.

Component: Rehmannia, mannitol, vitamine A, β-sitosterol.

Pharmacology: Protection of glycogen of liver, decreation of blood suger, refining contraction of cardiac muscle and circulation, elimination of fungus.

KING HERB	PIN YIN	熟地黄 SHU DI HUANG
君 药	LATIN	Radix Rehmanniae Praeparata
	ENGLISH	Prepared Adhesive Rehmannia Root
	GERMAN	Zubereitete Wurzel v. Rehmannia Glutinosa

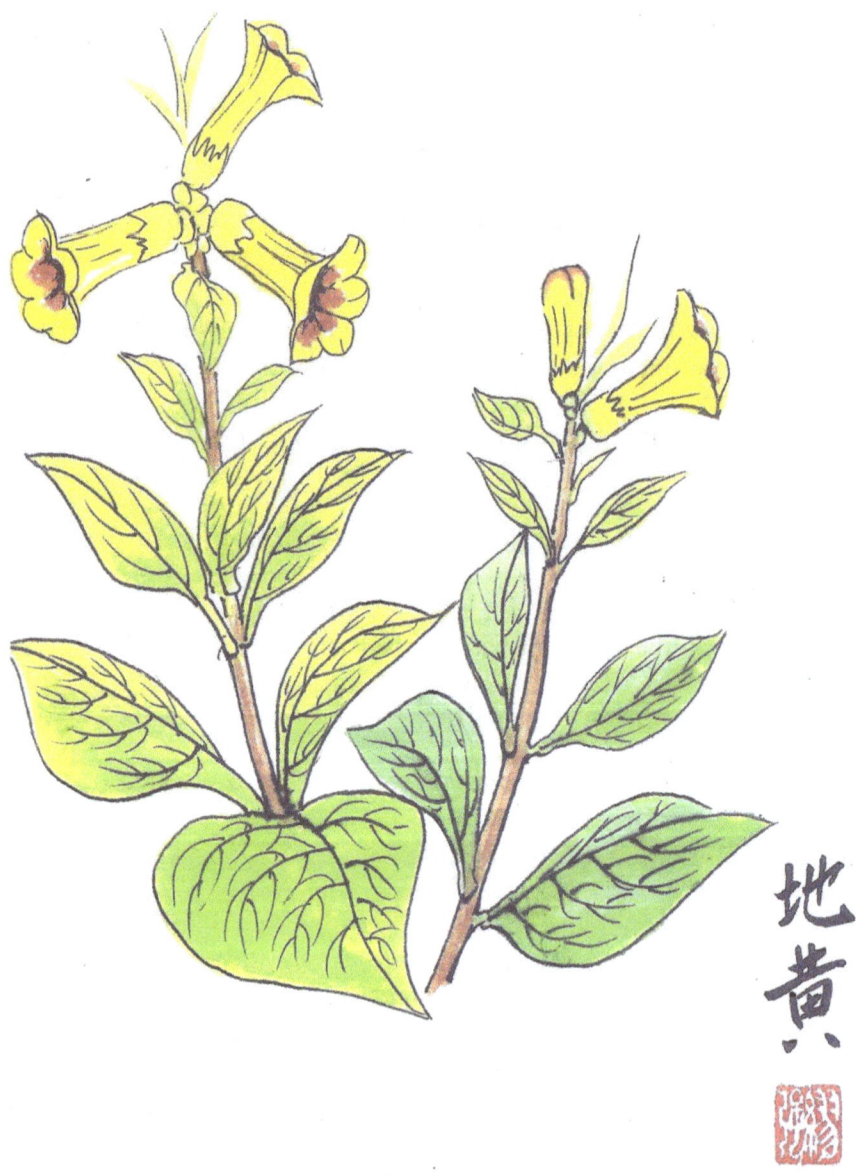

Fig. 43 Shu Di Huang

150

B. Blood warm and blocked, Qi weakness due to Yin deficiency

Long period of cirrhosis induces Yin deficiency of spleen, liver and kidney. The "Deficiency Fire" consumed itself fluid interior, Yang of spleen is weak, then Healthy Qi is deficiency, the blood is blocked, the water and moisture are stopped and gathered in the body, at least the ascites of abdomen is happened. At same time due to blood is heat, spitting blood and hemorrhage from nose and mouth appear. Owing to blood blocked, there would be vascular spider and blood texture in the face, chest and back with red spots and cinnabar palms. The swollen abdomen likes as dram, varicosis on abdominal wall is seriously, chest pain is sharply and subcostal stasis is hard, the face with black and yellow colors, heart and spirit are vexing.

The differentiation of above kinds of syndromes is "long time of ill damaged Yin of organ, blood and fluid". It is more difficult for therapy than situation of "A. Damage and Deficiency of Kidney Yang". In curing at first the herb of Huang Qi, Dang Gui are used to tonify Qi and reinforce Blood, Niu Xi and Bai Shao invigorate liver, at same time Fu Ling, Yin Chen and Ze Xie drain water and eliminate swollen. This means **"For draining water, reinforcing body's Qi must be done at first, when body's Qi flows fluently, water will be drained automatically."**

Case

Name: Lu, M. 62. Thirsty and more drinking are delayed for 9 years, abdominal distension has been for 9 months, abdominal circumference is 90cm, two legs has been swollen to the knee for 5 months. Patient was admitted in hospital in March 1992.

Laboratory Test: blood sugar: 22.4 mMol/L, albumin: 22g/L, globulin: 37g/L, creatinine: 72.5 µMol/L, urea nitrogen: 8.10 mMol/L.

Diagenosis of West Medicine: ascites due to cirrhosis, diabetes II, diabetic kidney disease.

Diagenosis of Chinese Medicine: tongue coating: light yellow, tongue texture: red, pulse: thready and wiry.

Disease Name of TCM: Shui Gu (水臌), Xiao Ke (消渴 Diabetes)。

Differentiation and Cure: Due to disease of diabetes, Qi and Yin are not enough, Qi blocked and blood detained, after long period of disease, liver and spleen are double

damaged. The evil of moisture blocked, the body's Qi of liver detained, water and moisture condensed and stopped.

Cure: tonifying Qi and activating blood, reinforcing Yin and eliminating heat, transporting and conducting water.

The recipe of herbs

中文	PIN YIN	LATIN	ENGLISH	GERMAN	Dosage,g
黄芪	Huang Qi	Astragali	Yellow Milk-Vetch	Astragaluswurzel	30
太子参	Tai Zi Shen	Radix Pseudostellariae	Prince Ginseng Root	Pseudostellariawurzel	30
石斛	Shi Hu	Herba Dandrobii	Dandrobium	Dandrobium	30
丹参	Dan Shen	Miltiorrhizae	Red Sege Root	Salvia-Wurzel	30
赤芍	Chi Shao	Paeoniae Rubrae	Red Peony Root	Pfingstrosewurzel	12
马鞭草	Ma Bian Cao	Herba Verbenae	Vervain	Eisenkraut	15
厚补	Hou Bu	Magnoliae	Magnolia Bark	Magnolienrinde	12
枳壳	Zhi Qiao	Fructus Anrantii	Orange Fruit	Orange	9

木香	Mu Xiang	Saussureae	Costus Root	Echte Kostwurzel	9
猪苓	Zhu Ling	Sclerotium Polypori	Polyporus Sclerotium	Porling	15
山楂	Shan Zha	Fuctus Crataegi	Hawthron Unripe Fruit	Frühe Fliederweiβ dornbeeren	15
鸡内金	Ji Nei Jin	Gigeriae Galli	Chicken Gizard Lining	Hünermagenendothel	9
车前草	Che Qian Cao	Herba Plantaginie	Plantago	Asiatisches Wegerichkraut	30

In this recipe Huang Qi and Tai Zi Shen are for tonifying Qi, Shi Hu is for reinforcing Yin, Dan Shen and Chi Shao are for activating blood, Hou Bu and Shan Za are for conducting Qi and descending adverse-raising Qi, the others are for clearing heat of blood and conducting water.

After 15 doses drunkings of this recipe, the urine amount per day reached about 2300 ml. Then the recipes were plused or reduced some herbs according the symptoms of patient, after drunk 12 dosages the circumference of abdomen was from 90cm decreased to 78cm, total protein was increased from 59g to 72g, albumin: globulin was 1:1. The patient was recovery.

**This case and recipe are from Prof. Yang, Ji Sun, Hang Zhou, China.

C. Double Deficiency of Body's Qi and Blood

For a long time of liver disease, the liver, splenn and kidney all are deficient, Qi and Blood are grand deficient also. There are either execess of stasis of phlegm and blood, or the deficiency of Qi and Blood. Generally, the patients have follows syndroms: abdominal distension with stuffiness and fullness, cardia palmus, breathe shortness, Face sallow and yellow, poor appetite, stool watery and thin, legs and abdomen swollen, amenia.

Case

Name: Ning, W. 38. first visiting in 1965. Abdominal circumference was 160cm, body weight was 85kg, varicosis on abdominal wall, In the last 10 years many times of intraperitoneal drainages were treated.

Diagnosis of West Medicine: Ascites due to cirrhosis.

Diagnosis of Chinese Medicine: tongue texture smooth, no coating, pulse: deep, thready and slowly.

Name in Chinese Medicine: Shui Gu (水臌).

Differentiation and Cure: double deficiency of Qi and Blood, water and moisture blocked. Tonifying Qi, reinforcing and activating Blood are the main method of therapy.

The recipe of herbs

中文	PIN YIN	LATIN	ENGLISH	GERMAN	Dosage,g
黄芪	Huang Qi	Astragali	Yellow Milk-Vetch	Astragaluswurzel	60
党参	Dang Shen	Radix Codonopsitia	Asiabell Root	Glockenwindenwurzel	10
当归	Dang Gui	Angelicae	Tangkuei	Chi. Angelika	10
赤芍	Chi Shao	Paeoniae Rubrae	Red Peony Root	Pfingstrosewurzel	10
白芍	Bai Shao	Paeoniae	White Peony	Weißepfingstrose	10
泽兰	Ze Lan	Lycopi Lucidi	Bugleweed	Wolfstrappkraut	10
红花	Hong Hua	Carthami Tinctorii	Safflower	Saflorblüten	10
桃仁	Xing Ren	Semen Persicae	Peach Seed	Pfirsichsamen	10

丝瓜络	Si Gua Luo	Fosciculus Vascularis Luffae	Dried Skeleton of Luffa Sponge	Luffa-Schwamm	10
茜草	Qian Cao	Rubiae	Modder	Krapp	15
通草	Tong Cao	Medula Tetrapanacis Popyriferi	Rice Paper Pith	Mark des Reispapierbaums	3
泽泻	Ze Xie	Rhizoma Alismatis Orientalitis	Water Plantain Rhizome	Orient-Froschlöffelknolle	10
车前子	Che Qian Cao	Semen Plantaginie	Seed Plantago	Asiatisches WEgerichsamen	15
抽葫芦	Chou Hu Lu	Trigonellae Foeni-Graeci	Fenugreek	Bockshornklee	15
鲜水葱	Xian Shui Cong	Allii Fistulosi	Green Onion	Winterzwiebel	30

Due to this patient has been ill for ten years, in this recipe a big amount of **Huang Qi has been used, maximum to 420g to tonify Qi.** With Dang Shen, Dang Gui and Bai Shao to be the "Minister Herbs", the healthy Qi and blood could be reinforced, the Blood would be actived. The above four kinds of herbs are given consideration in the differentiation for Yin-Yang: Qi-Blood and spleen-stomach. The other herbs are effective for eliminating moisture, conducting water, activating blood, resolving stasis, smoothing liver and regulating Qi. After 2 months theraphy, abdominal circumference of patient reduced to 80cm. The liver and spleen were not touched. Patient recovered healthy.

In the period of curing, only one time of intraperitoneal drainage was adopted, at same time a big amount of herbs of Huang Qi was used.

**This case and recipe are from Prof. Guan, You Bo, Beijing, China.

7.6. Hepatocarcinoma

Hepatocarcinoma is one of the commonly encountered cancer, the mortality is very high, from discovering the cancer to death, the survival time is generally about one month to one-year, average half year. Great majority of liver cancer is due to non-healing propagation of chronic hepatitis, or unsuccessful therapy, some times owing to carcinogen, such as nitrosaminc, aflatoxin, etc. Excessive drinking of alcohol, over tired and long time depression also be the causes.

The Chinese medical name of hepatocarcinoma is "Xue Gu (血臌)".

7.6.1. The causes and Mechanism of disease

The patient has gotten chronic hepatitis over a long time, Body's Qi detained and the blood blocked, the function of organs is declined, the healthy Qi is exhausted. Stasis of blood joints with phlegm and then is fested, the tumor develops quickly, the canceration appears.

In the period of invasion of hepatitis, some patients don't pay attention to cure; some of them is absentminded; some is drinking with big amount of alcohol, some is sadness, etc. They all miss an opportunity of best time of therapy and rehabilitation. At least cancer appeared.

7.6.2. Cure and Differentiation

According the thinking of Wholism therapy of TCM and the principle of "reinforcing body's Qi and eliminating evil Qi of pathogen", the patient is diagnosed by "Four Diagnosis" (inspection of vitality, listening and smelling, inquire, pulse), and the syndromes are differentiated with "Eight Differentiation" (Yin-Yang, Interior - Exterior, Deficiency- Excess, Cold-Warm). The

156

curing would be paid attention to "different patients with different syndromes and different recipes".

As soon as the patients are made definite diagnose of hepatocarcinoma, it is sure that all the patients have been deficiency of original Qi seriously already, and immunity decreased seriously also. In this time reinforcing healthy Qi is extremely important which includes: Regulating and tonifying spleen, liver and kidney, tonifying Qi and Blood, regulating body fluids to increase immunity to restrain, transform and perish the cells of cancer. On the side of eliminating evil Qi of pathogenesis, it is possible to use the herbs for antipyretic, detoxicate, resolving phlegm and stasis, realizing smoothing carthasising liver, such as Shan Ci Gu, Gua Lou, Bei Mu, Cao He Che, etc. It is forbidden absolutely to use the herbs of attacking and resolving stasis strongly. Otherwise the cancer will be promoted to proliferation of cancer.

Spleen and stomach are the postnatal basis of body, if the running of them is better, the healthy Qi and Blood will be produced, it is possible for remove phlegm blocks, softening stasis and resolving stagnation. The follows herbs could be used, Huo Xiang, Cang Shu, Shan Yao, etc. The famous Dr. Li, Dong Yuan (A.D.1180-1251) in his works 《Illustration of Spleen and Stomach 脾胃论》said, "The life still lives when there is Qi in stomach" and "Normal function of digestion means Life".

To therapy for liver cancer it's necessary to pay attention to activating Blood, resolving stasis, softening blocks and eliminating phlegm, after then the cancers will be smaller automatically. The herbs of Dang Gui, Chi Shao, Bai Shao, Dan Shen can tonify blood and reinforce healthy Qi.

Case

Name: Peng, M. 59. First visiting in Oct. 1991. Before 20 years the patient used to suffer from hepatitis, after treatment the function of liver was normal. In recent three months the follows syndromes appeared: acratia of total body, pain in chest, poor appetite, watery and thin of stool. Weight: 57.5 kg.

Laboratory test: TTT: 8, HbsAa: +, HbeAb: +, HbcAb: (+), AFP: 380µg /L. CT scanner: 10cm x 9.6cm x 8cm tumor edge unclear, behind right lobe of liver, CT Volume: 15 -44.2 Hu.

West Medical Diagnosis: Massive Hepatocarcinoma (right lobe).

Chinese Medical Inspection: Withered face with sallow color, tongue coating: white, pulse: deep and slippery.

Differentiation: Body's Qi is deficiency and Blood is blocked, phlegm and stasis stagnated permanently and jointed into mass

Chinese Medical Diagnose: Xue Gu (血臌).

Cure: Tonifying Qi and reinforcing healthy essence, activating blood and eliminating stasis, softening mass and resolving block.

The recipe of herbs

中文	PIN YIN	LATIN	ENGLISH	GERMAN	Dosage,g
党参	Dang Shen	Radix Codonopsitis	Asiabell Root	Glockenwindenwurzel	15
柴胡	Chai Hu	Radix Bupleuri	Thoroxax Root	Chi. Hasenohr	10
白术	Bai Shu	Rhizoma Macrocephalae Atractylodis	Largrhead White Atractylodes	Großköpftig Atractylodes	10
仓术	Cang Shu	Rhiroma Atroctylodis	Atractylodes	Atractylodes	10
旋复花	Fu Xuan Hua	Flos Inulae	Elecampane	Alantblüten	10
白芍	Bai Shao	Paeoniae	White Peony	Weißepfingstrose	10

砂仁	Sha Ren	Amomi	Grains-Paradise	Amomum-Sharen	10
茯苓	Fu Ling	Poriae Cocos	Hoelen	Kokospil	15
山慈菇	Shan Ci Gu	Pseudobulbus Shancigu	Chi. Tulip Bulb	Chi. Tulpenzwiebeln	10
川续断	Chuan Xu Duan	Radix Dipsaci Asperi	Teasel Root	Chi. Kardenwurzel	10
薏苡仁	Yi Yi Ren	Lachrymajodis	Job's Tears	Hiobstränen	10
山药	Shan Yao	Radix Dioscoreae	Chi. Wild Yam	Yamswurzelknollen	10

After took this recipe for two months, the test of CT scanner: tumor becomes smaller as 5cm x 5cm. AFP: 18.3 µg /L. After three months cure, AFP: 13.9 µg/L, Five months later (March 1992), CT scanner: 5cm x 4cm, edge clear and sharply. The patient's appetite increased much more, with red and smooth face, merry emotion. Weight increased to 62.5 kg. Now the situation of illness continuously takes favourable turn (2007).

**This case and recipe are from Prof. Guan, You Bo, Beijing, China.

7.7. Hepatonecrosis and Hepatic Coma

Generally speaking the causes of hepatonecrosis are toxicosis of pharmacy or food, for women some times owing to acute fatty liver in the period of gestation. This disease develops quickly and terriblely, the prognosis is very bad, the mortality is about 85%.

In Chinese medicine the name of hepetonecrosis is called "Ji Huang (急黄). 《Jin Kui Yao Lue (金匮要略)》 said, "The disease of Ji Huang is within a period of 18 days, full recovered in 10 days means lucky; otherwise the disease will be cured difficultly."

In clinic manifestation within 10 days of invasion there are follows syndromes of deep icterus, ascites, hemorrhage, coma and exhaust of kidney function, which is called "Acute Hepatonecrosis"; within 10 -50 days appearing above syndromes is called "Subacute Hepatonecrosis"; after 50 days is called "Chronic Hepatonecrosis".

7.7.1. Disease Causes and Mechanism

Hepatonecrosis is owing to moisture, heat and toxin are spread all over the "San Jiao (三焦)" , the fire of toxin attacks heart, Qi and blood are deficiency, Yin and Yang are all damaged, phlegm and moisture cover the spirit.

7.7.2. Differentiation and Cure

Hepatonecrosis is a severe hepatitis, its invasion develops very violently and quickly, coma and crisis appear, the situation is seriously danger. Facing the two sides of therapy: reinforcing healthy Qi and eliminating evil pathogenic Qi, it is very important to control the scale of herbs in recipe. If eliminating evil of pathogenic Qi be the main side of cure method and the reinforcing Qi is ignored, it's false absolutely that the Healthy Qi is exhausted, the patient dead instantly, doctors will lose the rescue opportunity. The most important for patient is maintaining the Qi and Blood, When the Qi and Blood still be existed in body of patient only, reinforcing the fire of Ming Men (Life Gate, 命门), rescure in the unseen world, there would be the possibility to take a turn better and be out of danger. In the moment of hundredweight hanging by a hair, the doctors should control the yardstick of herbs adopted in the recipe. With the principle that reinforcing Qi is the first and resolving evil pathogenic Qi is auxiliary, curing differentiate must be precisely, then rescue could bring the dying patient back to life.

Case 1

Name: Liu, W. 27. On 04, Feb. 1962, the patient suddenly pain seriously in the up abdomen with follows symptoms: yellow sclera, suggillation of total body, body temperature: 40 0 C, high fever continually, unconscious, stertorous breathing, swollen of four

160

limbs, grey stool and light-yellow urine, hemorrhage in vagina (before 100 days the patient admitted in another hospital for gestation and childbirth).

On 15, Feb. 1962 the patient was mis-diagnosed as cholelithiasis, and used to be operated in deep abdomen.

On 17, Feb. 1962 admitted to our hospital.

Laboratory Test: Icteric Index: 125, Bilirubin: 222.3μMol /L, TFT++, CCFT+++, ALT: 320U/L, Prothrombin Time (PT): 27 min, Non-Protein Nitrogen (NPN): 150mg/ dl, Hemokalemia:14.1 mg/ dl, Hemonatremia; 301.5 mg/ dl, Chloride: 250mg /dl, Leukocyte: 16600/ ml, Neutrality: 0.85, Basophil: 0-0.01, Limphocyte: 0.14.

West Medicine diagnosis: Acute infective icterohepatitis, Hepatic Coma, Septicemia, Acute Renal Function Failure, Azotemia.

Chinese Medicine diagnosis: Tongue coating: yellow, thick and greasy. Tongue texture: thin and pale. Pulse: extremely weak.

Chinese Medical Name of Illness: Ji Huang (急黄).

Differentiation: The evil Qi of moisture and heat damaged Liver and Gallbladder, and spread in "San Jiao" (breast and abdomen), covered the heart and spirit, the essence Qi of life will be disappeared, the crisis appeared.

Cure Principle: Tonifying Yin and Returning Yang, reinforcing essence Qi and Rescuing life, Stanching Bleeding and resolving stasis, eliminating moisture, clearing spirit and opening meridian.

The recipe of herbs

中文	PIN YIN	LATIN	ENGLISH	GERMAN	Dosage,g
西洋参	Xi Yang Shen	Radix Panacis Quinquefolli	American Gingseng	Amerikanische Kraftwurzel	9
侧柏炭	Ce Bai Tan	Cacumen Biotae Orientails	Burnt Arborvitae Leafy Twig	Verkohlte Orientalische Lebensbaumtriebspitzen	9
阿胶	E Jiao	Corii Asini	Ass Skin Glue	Eselshaut-Gelatine	9
地榆炭	Di Yu Tan	Radix Sanguisorbae	Burnt Bumet-Bloodworm Root	Verkohlte Wiesenknopwurzel	9
茵陈	Yin Chen	Artemisiae Scopariae	Virgate Wormwood	Besenbeifußkraut	15
黄连炭	Huang Lian Tan	Rhizoma Coptidis	Burnt Coptis Rhizome	Verkohlte Goldfadenwurzelstock	5
白芍	Bai Shao	Radix Paeonae	White Peony Root	Weißpfingstrose	30
当归	Dang Gui	Radix Angelicae	Red Sage Root	Chi. Angelikawurzel	12
生地黄	Sheng Di Huang	Rhizoma Rehmanniae	Fresh Chi. Foxlove Root	Frische Rehmanniawurzel	9
生甘草	Sheng Gan Cao	Radix Glycyrrhizae	Liquorice Root	Ural-Süßholz-Wurzel	5
金银花	Jin Yin Hua	Flos Lonicerae	Honeysuckle Flower	Heckenkirschblüten	30
麦冬	Mai Dong	Tuber Ophiopogonis	Greeping Lily-Turf Tuber	Schlanrenbartknollen	15
茯苓	Fu Ling	Sclerotium Poriae Cocos	Hoelen	Kokospilz	15
藕节	Ou Jie	Nodus Nelumbinis	Lotus Rezome Node	Lotusrizomknoten	9
紫肉桂	Zi Rou Gui	Cortex Cinnamomi Cassiae	Cinnamon Bark	Cassia-Zimtrinde	1.5
藿香叶	Huo Xiang Ye	Herb Pogostemonis	Cablin Patchouli	Patchoulikraut	3
胆草炭	Dan Cao Tan	Radix Gentianae Longdancao	Burnt Chi. Gentian Root	Verkohlte Chi. Enzianwurzel	9

162

After drank two doses of above recipe on 19, Feb. the patient recovered the spirit, stop snoring, hemorrhage smaller, the yellow color moved out from body. But the patient still not left the period of danger and crisis.

Plus, herbs of Dang Shen and Fu Long Gan in above recipe, the patient took drinking to 23, Feb., the hemorrhage stop, all the icterus has been disappeared, the spirit became clear. But the patient spoke still not clear and fluently, and was slow in reaction.

Laboratory Test: Icteric Index: 52U, Bilirubin: 30.78 µMol/ L, NPN: 29mg /dl.

Even if evil Qi of heat and moisture has been moved out, the healthy Qi of the patient was still lack, the second recipe has been adopted as follows.

The second recipe:

中文	PIN YIN	LATIN	ENGLISH	GERMAN	Dosage, g
西洋参	Xi Yang Shen	Radix Panacis Quinquefolli	American Gingseng	Amerikanische Kraftwurzel	5
茵陈	Yin Chen	Artemisiae Scopariae	Virgate Wormwood	Besenbeißkraut	30
白芍	Bai Shao	Radix Paeoniae	White Peony Root	Wei β e Pfingstrosewurzel	30
苍术	Cang Shu	Rhizoma Atroctylodis	Atractylodes	Atravtylodes	9
白术	Bai Zhu	Rhizoma Macrocephalae Atractylodis	Largrhead White Atractylodes	Großköpftig Atractylodes	9
茯苓	Fu Ling	Poriae Cocos	Hoelen	Kokospilz	15
杏仁	Xing Ren	Semen Pruni	Apricot Seed	Bittere Aprikosensamen	9
橘红	Ju Hong	Citri Erythrocarpae	Red Tangerine Peel	Rote Mandarinenschale	9

石斛	Shi Hu	Herba Debdrodium	Dendrobium Stem	Dendrobium	15
金银花	Jin Yin Hua	Flos Lonicerae	Honeysuckle Flower	Heckenkirsch Blüten	30
钩藤	Gou Teng	Ramulus cum Uncis Uncariae	Gambir vine Stem and Hooks	Uncariazweige und -Dornen	7.5
僵蚕	Jiang Can	Bombyx Batryticatus	Dead Stiff Body of Sick Silkworm Larvae	Tode Seidenspinnerraupen	3
石菖蒲	Shi Chang Pu	Rhizoma Acori Graminei	Sweetflag Rhizome	Acorus-Wurzelstock	9
牡丹皮	Mu Dan Pi	Cortex Moutan	Tree Peony Root bark	Strauchpaeonienwurzelrinde	9
天门冬	Tian Men Dong	Tuber Asparagi Cochinchinensis	Chinese Asparagus Tuber	Chinesische Spargelwurzel	9
麦门冬	Mai Men Dong	Tuber Ophiopogonis	Greeping Lily-Turf Tuber	Schlangenbartknollen	9
川贝母	Chuan Bai Mu	Bulbus Fritillariae Cirrhosae	Tendrilled Fritillary Bulb	Szechuan-Schachblumenzwiebel	12
紫花地丁	Yi Hua Di Ding	Herba cum Radice Violae Yedoensitis	Viola	Wildes Chinesisches Veilchen	15
藿香叶	Huo Xiang Ye	Herb Pogostemonis	Cablin Patchouli	Patchoulikraut	4.5

After taking 5 doses of this recipe, the patient has recovered health basically. Then removing out Xi Yang Shen in this recipe, the patient continuously took some doses of above recipe and recovered healthy totally and left hospital.

164

Analysis of this Case 1

In this case the disease is acute infectional icterohepatitis originally, but the clinic manifestation was similar as biliary tract obstruction with concurrent infection. Then the operation was fault as biliary tract problem and promotes the situation of the patient worsened. The operation conducted the acute failure of liver and kidney. The follows syndromes appeared: uremia, hepatitis coma, electrolyte disorder, memorrhage widely, septismia. State of illness is very serious.

From the differentiation, this disease is due to the evil of moisture and heat held and hid in liver and gallbladder interior, and spread fully into San Jiao (三焦) , covered heart and spirit, the evil of heat invided into blood, and pressed blood running out of the vessels, the symptoms is seriously. Owing to Qi and Blood are double deficiency, the body's healthy Qi is exhausted. The phenomenon is exposed that the original Qi has disappeared nearly. Due to losing big amount of blood (haemorrhage: purpura of total body, passing blood in stool frequently, metrorrhagia), the Yin Blood became weakness and nearly disappeared, The Yang Qi can not adhere to the substance of blood, the pulse was very weak nearly to cut off, in an instant the patient is possible to death.

According the situation that Yang Qi would be removed out, the evil Qi was rampant, in curing we must give priority to reinforce and keep the only less body's Qi. Just maintaining healthy Qi, it's possible to eliminate the evil Qi. Conversely if to give priority to remove out the evil Qi, it's possible that the evil Qi could not be removed but the body's healthy Qi could be exhausted and the patient could be dead.

In the two above recipes, Xi Yang Shen and Mai Men Dong invigorate the Yin and recover the pulse. Sheng Di Huang, Dang Gui and Bai Shao tonify blood, Rou Gui reinforce the life fire of Ming Men (Life Gate). Ce Bai Tan, Di Yü Tan, Chuan Huang Lian Tan, Dan Cao Tan, Mu Dan Pi clear heat, cool blood and stanch bleeding. Yin Chen, Jin Yin Hua, Fu Ling and Huo Xiang conduct out moisture and detoxicate. Shi Chang Pu and Yuan Zhi open heart and spirit to relieve heat and moisture which covered the heart. These two herbs are only used for emergency.

There are not attaching and expelling herbs in the two receipts, it seems prosaic, but the herbs are conformity with the syndromes. After 2 doses drunk, the icterus began removed, the spirit became clear and hemorrhage stop gradually. After 6 doses drunk the icterus disappeared and bleeding stop, that means 70% of illness situation has been controlled. At this time the mantal activity didn't still recover, Dang Shen, Cang Shu and Bai Zhu can invigorate spleen and reinforce healthy Qi. To remove the herbs of cooling blood and stopping bleeding, increase the herbs of Chuan Bei Mu and Jü Hong to conduct Qi, which can open stomach and eliminate phlegm. Gou Teng and Jiang Can cool down liver, remove out spasm and detoxy.

In the rescue of about 20 days, the postmortem patient with critical mortality illness of acute hepatonecrosis and coma had recovered health and left hospital.

**This case and recipe are from Prof. Guan, You Bo, Beijing, China.

Case 2

Name: Miao, M. 64, on 02, Jul.2006 sudden attacked by acute hepatonecrosis with black jaundice, total skin of body and face were with deep yellow and black colour, urine was black. Patient felt very tired. Laboratory test on 07, Jul.: GOT: 2.280, GPT: 1596, Bilirubin: 27.18. On 08, Jul. the patient took the follows recipe 1 of Chinese herbs (4 doses) by Dr. Xiong, Chun Jin. After 4 days, labor. test: GOT: 247, GPT: 706, Bilirubin: 28.30.

The recipe 1 q

中文	PIN YIN	LATIN	ENGLISH	GERMAN	Dosage,g
茵陈	Yin Chen	Artemisiae Scopariae	Virgate Wormwood	Besenbeißkraut	30
金钱草	Jin Qian Cao	Herb Lysimachiae	Christina Loosestrife	Felberich	20
乌梅	Wu Mei	Fructus Pruni Mume	Ume Plum Fruit	Umeaprikosenfrüchte	15
海金沙	Hai Jin Sha	Spora Lygodii	Climbing Fern Spore	Kletterfarnsporen	15
郁金	Yu Jin	Tuber Curicumae	Tumeric Tuber	Gelbwurzelknolle	15
生山查	Sheng Shan Zha	Fructus Crataegi	Hawthron Unripe Fruit	Frühe Fliederweiß dornbeeren	12
白术	Bai Zhu	Rhizoma Macrocephalae Atractylodis	Largrhead White Atractylodes	Großköpftig Atractylodes	10
赤勺	Chi Shao	Paeoniae Rubrae	Red Peony Root	Pfingstrosewurzel	10
柴胡	Chai Hu	Radix Bupleuri	Thorowax Root	Chi. Hasenohrwurzel	10
车前草	Che Qian Cao	Herba Plantaginie	Plantago	Asiatisches Wegerichkraut	10
五味子	Wu Wei Zi	Fuctus Schisandrae Chi.	Northern Schisandra Fruit	Schisandra-Früchte	6
刘寄奴	Liu Ji Nu	Herba Artemisiae	Artemisia	Schwefel	6
丹皮	Dan Pi	Fructus Crataegi	Hawthron Unripe FRuit	Frühe Fliederweiß dornbeeren	6

On 13, Jul. the patient was in one klinikum of a university in Germany. Acute hepatitis E and hepatonecrosis was diagnosed, and owing to nearly failure of function of liver doctors suggested the operation of liver transplant should be implemented, On 16, Jul. 2006, laboratory test suddenly turns better, GOT was falled down to 79, GPT to 361, Bilirubin is 28,70. Doctors and patient all agreed to take conservative treatment.

In the night of 22, Jul. the myocardial infarction happened and with headache, flusteredness and serious gasp, the pulse was about 110 /min. Oxygen inhalation was no effective. Doctors decided to do the contrast examination of coronary artery to detect whether the arterial is narrow and prepared the stents with balloon catheters. After the examination, dramatic result was shown that the arteries of coronary were normal as young man and no blocked (Fig. 44). Later several days the infarction was remittence automatically.

On 01, Aug. the syndromes of regurgitation of gastric juice and vomiting of gastric acid happened. From the test of gastroscopic observation, the scars ulcers and much more ulcer points on the tissue of stomach were discovered. (see fig. 45 gastroscopy) The patient was recovered after taking some medicines of stomach.

On 03, Aug. the terrible ascites of abdomen appeared which developed from feet to thigh and from hypogastric to epigastric zone. The circumference of abdomen increased from 75cm to 100cm and the weight of the body from 67kg to 90gk within two weeks. No abnormal tissues were discovered after the test of needle biopsy of liver,and the liver was 16cm length (no swollen) by ultrasonic test). The situation of illness developed critically.

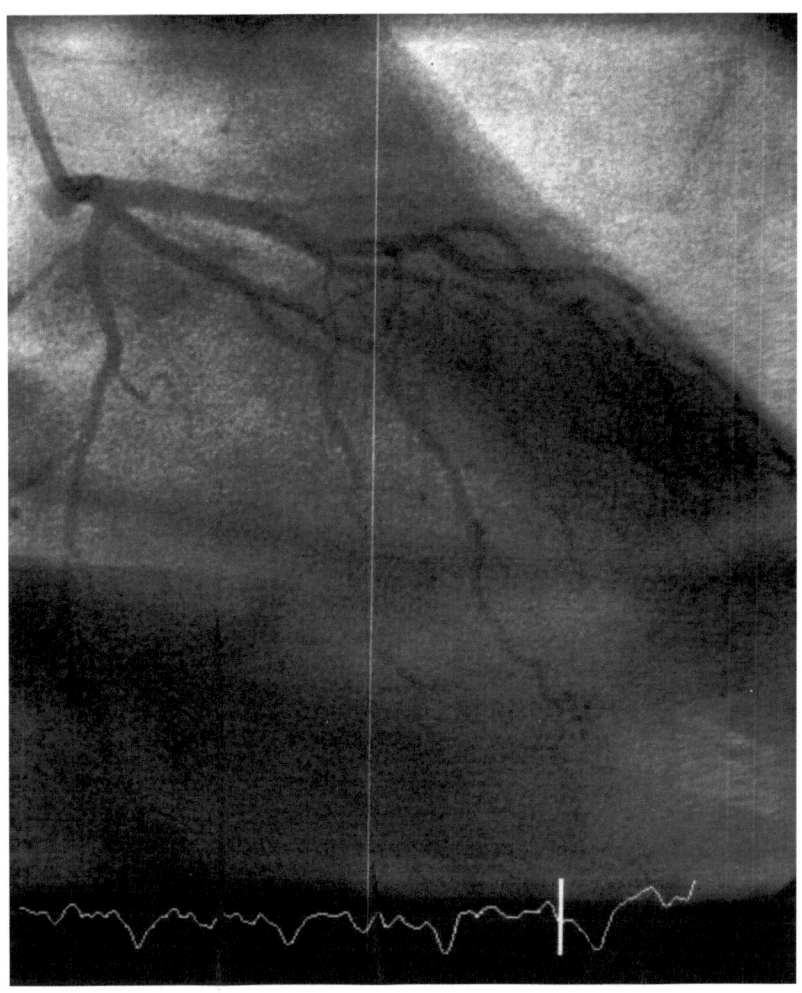

Fig. 44 Coronary arteriography

Some treatments were adopted and no effect, e.g. venous transfusion of hepatin, etc. The laboratory test on 07, Aug. is albumin: 25 g/L, globulin: 46g/L. At least doctor adopted decisive treatment, after the test of abdominoscope (with three perforations through abdominal wall and air pumping for floating of liver), the scars and damages on the surface of liver were discovered, that means before several ten years the patient has been suffered by hepatitis. From the memorial of patient before 20 years the pain at chest always happened but the laboratory test was normal.

After 30 bottles of plasma albumin (250ml / bottle) of intravenous injection, the situation was taken favourable turn: the amount of urine was 1000 ml per day average and maximum was 3200 ml one day. The ascites of abdomen disappeared gradually from up to lower abdomen and the swollen of legs scope reduced from thigh to shank and foot instep. The weight was recovered to 67kg and the circumference of abdomen reduced to 78 cm. The test on 14, Aug. is albumin: 36 g/L, globulin: 30 g/L. On 22, Aug. 2006 the patient left hospital and recovered healthy basically.

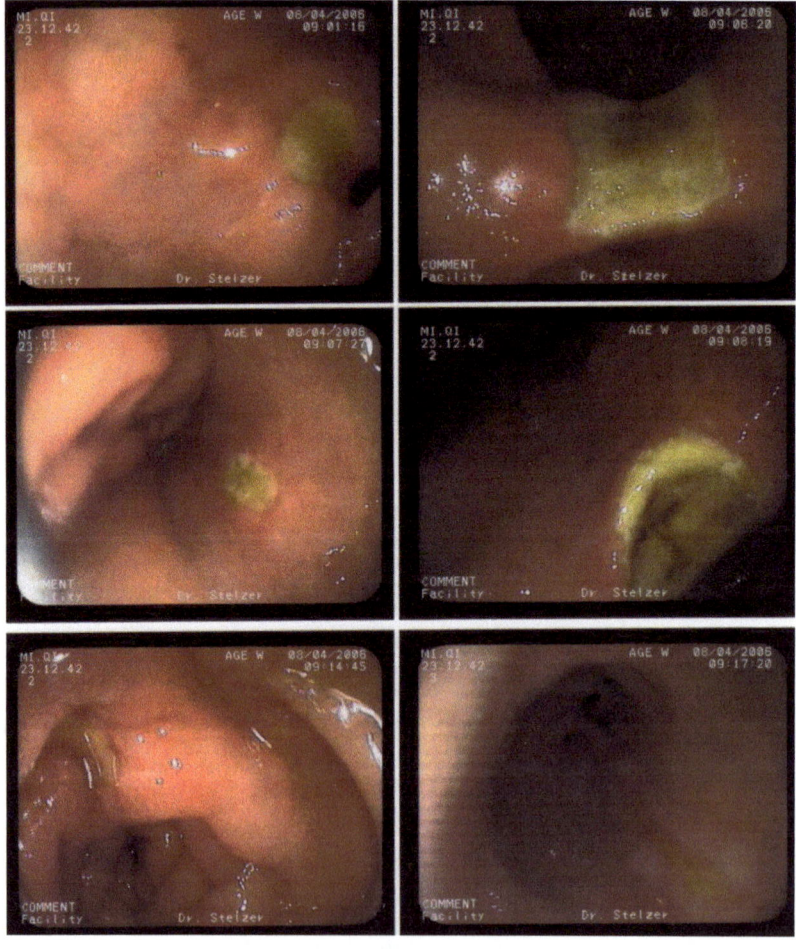

Fig. 45　Gastroscope

170

In late half year the patient took about the famous Chinese herbs recipe of "Xiao Chai Hu Tang 小柴胡汤" (by Dr. Zhang, Zhong Jing, Han Dynasty). In this receipt the front 3 herbs are purging the heat and moisture, the behind 3 herbs are tonic of Qi and Blood.

The recipe 2:

中文	PIN YIN	LATIN	ENGLISH	GERMAN	Dosage, g
柴胡	Chai Hu	Radix Bupleuri	Thorowax Root	Chi. Hasenohrwurzel	12
法半夏	Fa Ban Xia	Rhizoma Pinelliae Ternatae	Prepared Pinellia Rhizome	Vorbehandelte Pinellia Knollen	9
黄芩	Huang Qin	Radix Scutellariae Baicalensis	Baical Scullcap Root	Baikal-Helmkrautwurzel	9
大枣	Da Zao	Ziziphi Jujubbae	Chi. Black Date	Daeeelfrücht	4 pies.
干姜	GanJiang	Rhizoma Zingiberia	Dried Ginger	Getrochente Ingwer	9
甘草	Gan Cao	Radix Glycyrrhizae Preperata	Piquorice Root prepared	Ural-Süßholz-Wurzel Rösten	6

King Herb: Chai Hu, Radix Bupleuri (Fig. 46)

Flora: Carrot family, perennial, Herbacerous

Character: Bitter, Balance

Meridian: Perricardium, San Jiao, Liver, Gallbadder

Function: Catharsising liver, relieving depression, lifting Yang, relieving exterior syndroms and antipyretic.

Component: Volatile (buoleuumol), fatty oil, sterol, rutin, gledinin.

171

Pharmacology: Chai Hu has excellent function of antipyretic and detoxication. It can promote secrete of bile, eliminate fatty liver to protect liver and to increase immunity. It can also inhibit virus and bacteria. At last it promotes peristalsis of stomach and intestine and healing of ulcer of digestive canal.

This recipe has two functions, one is to catharsis the else heat and moisture in the liver and spleen; the second is to reinforce the Yin of organs. After taking about several dozens of above recipes of herbs, the patient recovered healthy better. The else swollen on instep has disappeared.

Recipe 3

中文	PIN YIN	LATIN	ENGLISH	GERMAN	Dosage ,g
熟地黄	Shu Di Huang	Rhizoma Rehmanniae	Prepared Chi. Foxlove Root	Verbehandelte Rehmanniawurzel	1 5
淮山药	Huai Shan Yao	Radix Dioscoreae Oppositae	Chi. WildYam Root	Yamswurzelknollen	20
茯苓	Fu Ling	Poriae Cocos	Hoelen	Kokospilz	10
丹皮	Dan Pi	Fructus Crataegi	Hawthron Unripe Fruit	FrüheFliederweißdornbeeren	10
泽泻	Ze Xie	Rhizoma Alismatis Orientalitis	Water Plantain Rezome	Orient-Froschlöffelknolle	10
山萸肉	Shan Yü Rou	Fructus Corni Officinalis	Dogwood Fruit	Knollekirschenfrüchte	15
天门冬	Tian Men Dong	Tuber Asparagi Cochinchinensis	Chinese Asparagus Tuber	Chi. Spargelwurzel	15

麦门冬	Mai Men Dong	Tuber Ophiopogonis	Greeping Lily-Turf Tuber	Schlangenbartknolle	15
益智仁	Yi Zhi Ren	Fructus Alpiniae Oxyphyllae	Black Cardamon Fruit	Alpinia-Früchte	10
桑寄生	Sang Ji Sheng	Ramulus Sangjisgeng	Mulberry Mistletoe Stem	Mistel oder Riemenblume	15
薏苡仁	Yi Yi Ren	Semen Coicis	Coix Seed	Hiobstränen Samen	15
杜仲	Du Zhong	Cortex Eucommiae	Eucommia Bark	Chi. Guttapercharinde	10
白芍	Bai Shao	Rezoma Paeoniae	White Peony Root	Weißepfingstrosewurzel	10
白芥子	Bai Jie Zi	Semen Sinapis Albae	White Mustard Seed	Weiße Senfknörner	6
甘草	Gan Cao	Radix Glycyrrhizae	Liquorice Root	Ural-Süβholz-Wurzel	6

On 06, Nov. 2006, Dr. Chun-Jin Xiong wrote the second recipe as above Recipe 3

This recipe is for the long-time ill patient to recover the physical power. Shu Di Huang, Huai Shan Yao and Yi Zhi Ren are tonifying Yin of kidney. Fu Ling, Dan Pi, Shan Yu Rou, Ze Xie and Yi Yi Ren are regulating and reinforcing the Yin of spleen organ. Sang Ji Sheng, Du Zhong are tonifying Yin of liver. Tian Men Dong, Mai Men Dong and Bai Jie Zi are reinforcing the Yin of lunge. Bai Shao is regulating and activating the blood. In this recipe the King Herb is Shu Di Huang. The patient took about per ten doses of this recipe herbs in one year, and recovered the working capability of half day.

Before leafing hospital in August 2006, a 2cm granulation was discovered in the lungs' right side near the bronche with CT and biopsy test. With the better situation of healthy recovered, in the CT testing in April 2010 doctors found the granuloma disappeared automatically.

KING HERB	PIN YIN	柴胡 CHAI HU
	LATIN	Radix Bupleuri
君　药	ENGLISH	Chinese Thorowax Root
	GERMAN	Chinesische Hasenohrwurzel

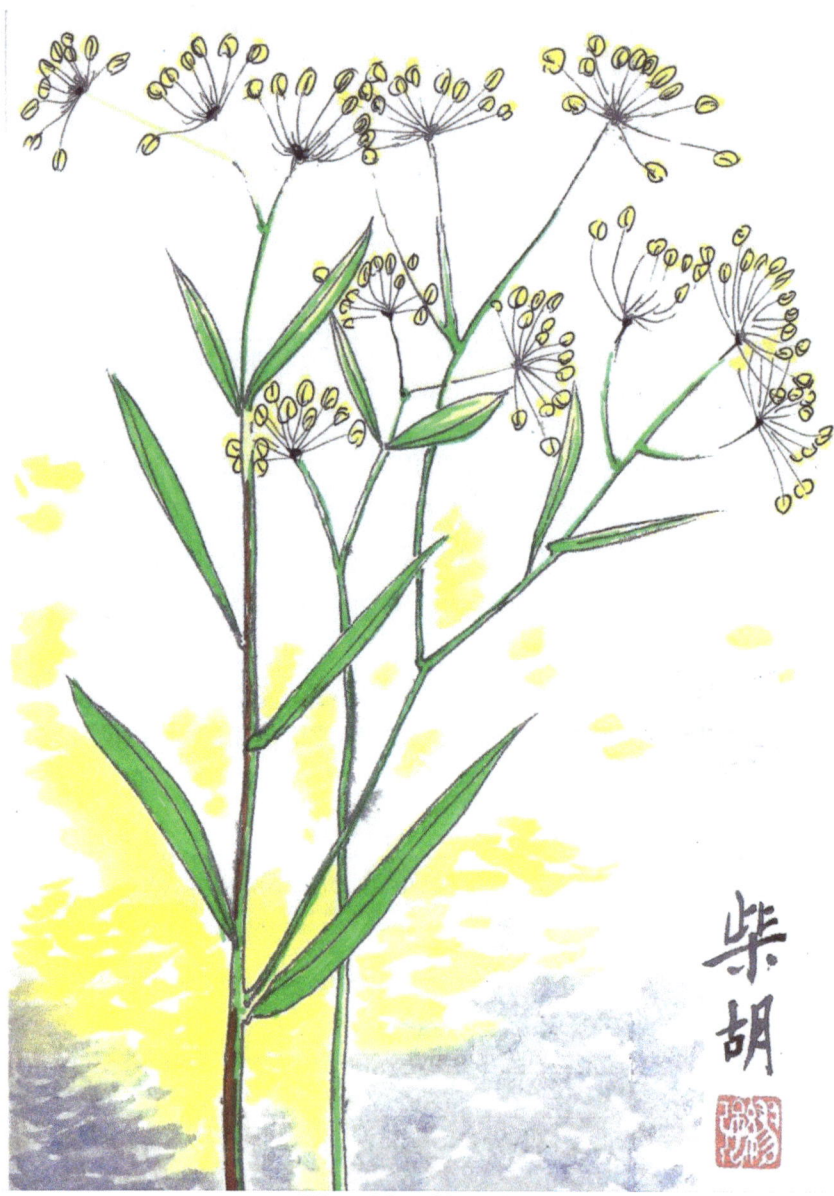

Fig. 46   Chai Hu

The Analysis of the Differentiation of Case 2

Date	Syndrom	Wu Xing Analysis	Differentiation and Therapy
2,7,2006	Hepatonecrosis Black Icterus Hemorrhage from nose	Wood(liver) attacked by heat and moisture, Earth (spleen), and Water (kidney) are weakness, can't support Wood. （水虚不能生木）	Receipt 1: Yin Chen, Jin Qian Cao and Hai Jin Sha remove out heat n moist and expell icterus. Yü Jin, Chi Shao activate and tonify blood, Liu Ji Nu is used for hemostasis. Wu Bei Zi reinforces liver and kidney.
22,07,06	Myocardial Infarction	Wood (liver) is weak, can not produce and reinforce Fire (Heart) （木弱不能生火）	Function of heart is weakness, but no organic demaged. When liver function is better, Myocardial Infarction disappears automaticly.
01,08,06	Vomiting gastric acid	Wood (liver) over controls Earth (spleen and stomach) (木乘土)	Failture of liver's function induces pathogenesis of stomach (gastric acid, duodenal and stomath ulcer).
03,08,06	Ascites happened and serious day and day	Water (Kidney, Mother)bears Wood (Liver,Son)when liver is too weak, so steals Mother's Qi (子盗母气) and then Kidney demaged and loses function of closing and opening of water tunnel.	Plasma albumin of intravenous injection tonifys Yin of blood, reinforces liver and kidney, ascites is disappeared.
20,80,06 16,04,10	Granulation of Lungs	Wood (Liver) anti-controls Metal (Lungs) (木悔金)	Take receipts 2 and 3 for three years continuously removed out moist and heat tonify liver, kidney and spleen, patient has recovered Qi and Blood, the granulation disappeared automatically. It means Earth bears Metal (土生金).

8. The Theraputical Operation of Acupuncture for Hepatitis

8.1. Icterohepatitis

8.1.1. The Causes of Icterohepatitis

A. The spleen and stomach are damaged by evil of moisture, digestion is blocked, stool and urine are astringed.

B. Over drinking of alcohol.

C. Over tired due to working.

D. Interior damaged by emotion, especially by over thinking and terror.

8.1.2. The Principle of Curing

A. The jaundice is divided into two kinds: "Yin Huang" (阴黄 Yin Jaundice) and "Yang Huang" (阳黄 Yang Jaundice). Yang Jaundice is induced by evil of heat and moisture, it is necessary to remove out heat, conduct moisture away and catharsis spleen. Yin Jaundice is due to cold and moisture, tonifying Qi, Yang of Blood and Spleen are necessary.

B. In curing pay attention to diaphoresis and conducting urine.

8.1.3. Differentiation and Cure

IN TCM from the syndromes, there are three kinds of icterohepatitis: Yang Jaundice, Yin Jaundice and "Yü Xüe Jaundice 淤血黄" (Blood Stasis Jaundice belongs to Yin Jaundice).

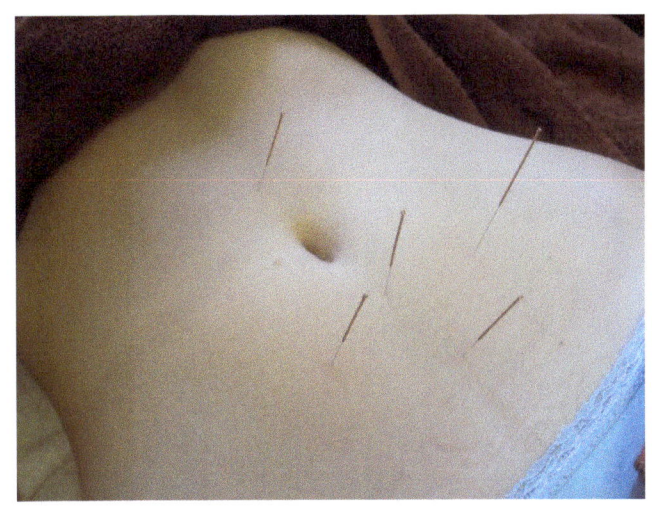

Fig. 47 Akupuncture

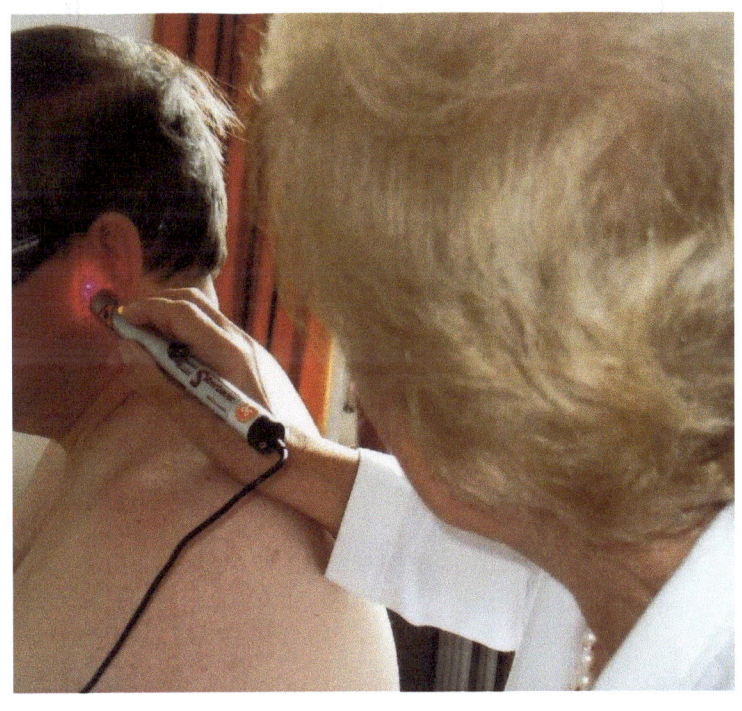

Fig. 48 Laser Akupuncture

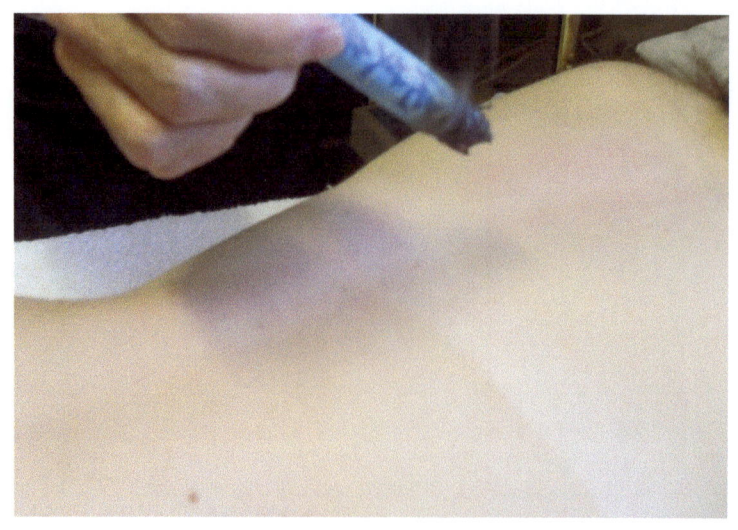

Fig. 49 Moxibastion

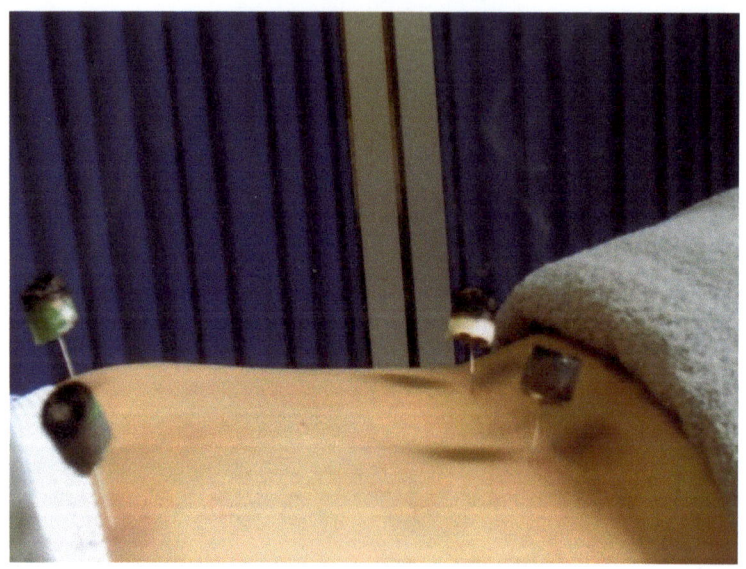

Fig. 50 Acupuncture plus Moxibustion

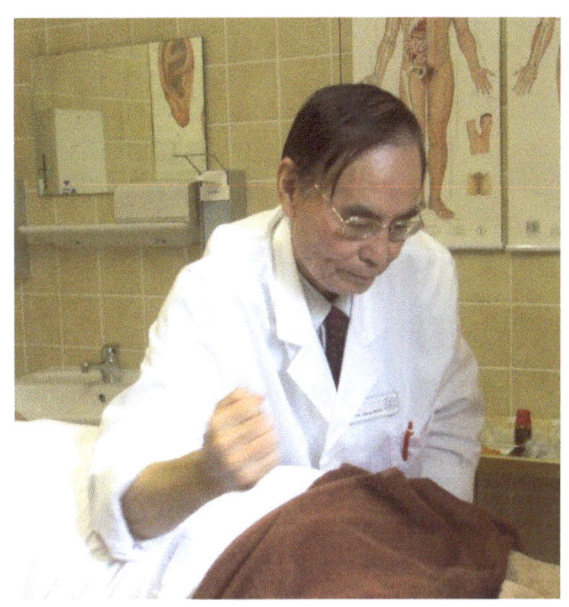

Fig. 51 Chinese Acu-Massage

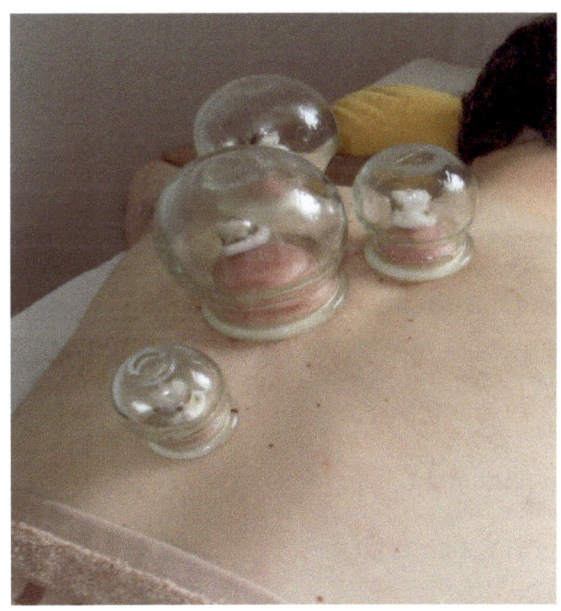

Fig. 52 Cupping

8.1.3.1. Yang Jaundice

A. Syndromes: vexing heat, thirst, polyorexia, stool and urine astringed, face and body with bright and yellow colour. Tongue coating: yellow and greasy, pulse: grand, slippery and surging.

B. Principle of Curing:

Relieving exterior, clearing heat, removing moisture out.

C. Meridian: Feet Shao Yang Gallbladder, Feet Jue Yin Liver, Feet Yang Ming Stomach, Feet Tai Yin Spleen.

Points: Dan Shu (DU 19), Zhong Feng (LI 4), Yang Ling Quan (GB 34), Nei Ting (ST 44), San Yin Jiao (SP 6). (see Fig. 48, 49, 50)

D, Manual Method: Catharsis.

E. Differentiation: Abdomen distention: plus Zhong Wan (RE 12). Vomit: plus Nei Guan (PC 6). Constipation: plus Da Chang Shu (BL 25).

8.1.3.2. Yin Jaundice

A. Syndromes: Feeling cold, liking silence, oppressed feeling in chest, poor appetite, stool: diarrhea and slippery, urine: thin and long, body and face with deep yellow color. Uncoated tongue, Pulse: deep and weak.

B. Principle of Curing:

Warming and regulating Yang of spleen.

C. Meridians and Points:

Meridian: Feet Taiyang Bladder, Feet Tai Yin Spleen, Feet Yang Ming Stomach.

Points: **Pi Shu (BL 20), Zhong Wan (Re 12). Gong Sun (SP 4), Zu San Li (ST 36), Ming Men (DU 4), Tian Shu (ST 25).**

D. Manual Method: Reinforcing style, with moxibustion.

8.1.3.3. Blood Stasis Jaundice

A. Syndromes: Face with black color, abdominal pain, some times masses in subcostal, stool and urine with black color, skin with yellow color, fever. Pulse: deep and irregular intermittent.

B. Principle of Curing: Breaking masses and generating vitality.

C. Meridians: Feet Tai Yang Bladder, Feet Tai Yin Spleen.

Points: Gan Shu (BL 18), Ge Shu (BL 17), San Yin Jiao (SP 6), Zhang Men (LI 13), Zhong Wan (RE 12).

D. Manual Method: Catharsis.

8.2. Chronic Hepatitis

The Chinese Medical name of chronic hepatitis is "Xie Tong 胁痛" （Chest Pain）. Syndromes: always pain in chest, some times seriously.

8.2.1. Cause of disease

A. After acute hepatitis, the evil Qi is still detained in liver and gallbladder, the illness is propagated with non-healing, Health Qi and Blood is blocked.

B. Grand anger happened and Qi adverse raises, hurried Qi and excessive fire are blocked in chest.

C. Due to long time illness, Liver and kidney became weakly, the function of activity of Qi and producing of Blood is disturbed.

D. Differentiation:

The differentiation must be divided in two situations: Exterior pathogenic factors and interior damagement.

(1) Pain owing to melancholy and fatigue: points of acupunture are adoped by Heart and Lunge meridian's points.

(2) Pain owing to food and drinking and over tired: adopting Spleen meridian and Stomach meridian's points.

(3) Over sexual intercourses and interior damaged (water tunnels blocked): adopting Kidney and Bladder meridian's points.

8.2.2. Principle of Curing

Catharsis, dissipating masses, activating Qi and blood.

A. Owing to exterior pathogenic factors: Reconciliation therapy is important. It's necessary to adopt Feet Shao Yang Gallbladder and Hand Shao Yang San Jiao meridian's points.

B. Owing to interior organ damaged: Cure should pay attention to liver and gallbladder, adopting Feet Jue Yin Liver meridian and Feet Shao Yang Gallbladder meridian's points.

8.2.3. Differentiation and Cure

The following 5 kinds of situations are commonly seen:

8.2.3.1. Invasion of pathogen of heat and moisture

A. Syndromes: Stuffiness and pain in chest, poor appetite, vomit, dizzy. Tongue coating: white and thin, Pulse: wiry.

B. Principle of curing: Reconciliation of liver and gallbladder.

C. Meridian: Feet Shao Yang Gallbladder meridian.

Points: Da Zhui (DU 14), Xia Xi (GB 43), Qi Men (LI 14), Nei Guan (PC 6).

D.Method: Balance between catharsis and tonic.

8.2.3.2. Excessive fire of Liver

A. Syndromes: Always anger, eyes swollen and pain, instability of spirit and emotion, dizzy, sharp pain in chest.

B. Principle of Cure: Clearing liver and catharsis of fire.

C. Meridian: Feet Jue Yin Liver and Feet Shao Yang Gallbladder meridian

Points: Tai Chong (LI 3), Xing Jian (LI 2), Xia Xi (GB 43), Zhi Gou (SJ 6).

D. Method: catharsis.

8.2.3.3. Melancholy and pain in chest

A. Syndromes: Absentminded, poor appetite, sign and tired always. Tangue coating: greasy and with pink color. Pulse: wiry.

B. Principle of curing: Catharsis of liver, resolving melanciliation.

C. Meridian: Feet Tai Yang Bladder, Feet Jue Yin Liver meridian and Ren Mai.

Points: Gan Shu (BL 18), Dan Shu (BL 19), Qi Men (LI 14), Zhong Wan (RE 12).

D. Method: catharsis.

8.2.3.4. Blood blocked and pain in chest

A. Syndromes: Pain continuously and with fixed location, much more pain when chest is pressed, eyes are with black color, skin is roughly and keratosis.

B. Principle of curing: resolving blocked blood.

C. Meridian: Hand Shao Yang San Jiao Meridian, Feet Jue Yin Liver meridian.

Points: Zhi Gou (SJ 6), Qi Men (LI 14), Ge Shu (BL 17), Tai Chong (LI 3).

D.Method: catharsis.

8.2.3.5. Deficiency of liver and pain in chest

A. Syndromes: Pain in chest and it is better when pressed, the two eyes seems to be seeing no thing, the body is weakness.

Tangue texture: thin and pale, Coating: white. Pulse: thready and wiry.

B. Priciple of curing: Tonicity of blood, reinforcing liver.

C. Meridian: Feet Shao Yin Kidney Meridian, Feet Tai Yang Bladder Meridian.

Points: Tai Xi (KI 3), Gan Shu (BL 18), Ge Shu (BL 17), Shen Shu (BL 23), Dan Shu (BL 19).

Method: reinforcement.

8.3. Hepatocirrhosis

Before 2500 years there had been the classification of hepatitis, including Acute infective icterohepatitis, chronic hepatitis, hepatocirrhosis, ascites, hepatocarcinoma and hepatic coma.

The Chinese Medical name of Hepatocirrhosis is "Zheng Jia 癥瘕". 《Zhu Bing Yuan Hou Lun 诸病源侯论》 (<Treatise on the Pathogenisis and Manifestation of Diseases>, Author: Chao, Yuan

184

Fang 巢元方, A.D. 610, China) appointed: " The mass unmoved is named Zhen (癥), moved by pushing is named Jia (瘕)".

A. The Cause of Hepatocirrhosis: Qi blocked and Blood detained. Melancholia

of seven emotion.

B. Principle of curing: activating blood and resolving stasis, reinforcing healthy Qi and softening mass.

C. Meridian: Feet Yang Ming Stomach Meridian, Feet Tai Yin Spleen Meridian,

Points: Zu San Li (ST 36), San Yin Jiao (SP 6), Zhong Wan (RE 12), Tian Shu (ST 25), Qi Hai (RE 6).

D. Method: catharsis or uniform of reinforcing and catharsis.

**The Chapter 8 are total from Prof. LIU, Han Yin 《 The Complete Volume on Practical Acupuncture 1988》

Chinese Dynasties

（from Huang Di to Qing Dynasty）

DYNASTY	朝代	Period
Huang Di	黄帝	v.c. 3000
Xia Dynasty	夏朝	v.c. 2100 – v.c. 1600
Shang Danasty	商朝	v.c. 1600 - v.c. 1100
Xi Zhou	西周	v.c. 1100 – v.c. 770
Dong Zhou	东周	v.c. 770 – v.c. 256
Chun Qiu (Spring Autumn)	春秋	v.c. 770 – v. c. 476
Zhan Guo (Warring States)	战国	v.c. 475 – v.c. 221
Qin Dynasty	秦朝	v.c. 221 – v.c. 207
Han Dynasty	汉朝	v.c. 206 – a.c. 220
San Guo (Three Kingdoms)	三国	220 -280
Xi Jin	西晋	265 – 316
Dong Jin	东晋	317 – 420
Nan Bei Chao	南北朝	420 -581
Sui Dynasty	隋朝	581 - 618
Tang Dynasty	唐朝	618 – 907
Five Danasties	五代	907 – 960
Song Dynasty	宋朝	960 – 1179
Yuan Dynasty	元朝	1271 – 1368
Ming Dynasty	明朝	1368 – 1644
Qing Dynasty	清朝	1644 - 1911

ILLUSTRATION

In compiling of chapters of "Traditional Chinese Medicine is Wholism Medicine", author consulted the book of "The Basic Theory of Chinese Medicine"Chief Editor: Prof. YIN Hui He）

Author consulted quated the differentiation and cases of hepatosis from the book of "The Analyze of Hepatosis cases by GUAN You Bo" (author: Prof. ZHAO Bo Zhi), and the book of "The Proven Receipts of Hepatosis by Famous and Senior Experts of TCM" (Editors: XU Jiang Yan, LIU Wen Li, YANG Jian Yu, DU Lai). In these two books, the cases and analysis finished by Prof. GUAN You Bo, ZHU Liang Chun, QIAO Bao Jun, LIU Du Zhou, WU Jun Yu, YANG Ji Sun, YAN De Xin and DAI Yu Guang, etc. are quoted and referred to.

In the chapter 8 of Acupuncture, author refer to the book of "The Complete Volume on Practical Acupuncture" (written by Prof. LIU Han Yin, Nov.1988) in which the chapters of Cure of Icterohepatitis, Chronic Hepatitis and Hepatocirrhose are quoted.

The component and pharmacology of herbs are referred to the book of "The Manual of Chinese Herbs in Clinic", Shanghai TCM College, Institute of Recipe and Herbs.

Fig. 14 is from the Experiment Report of "The Observation of Cytoskeleton Structure of the Epithelial Cell" (Author: WANG Bing Shui, FANG Heng Hu, REN Dong Qing) which is published in the book of "Foundation of Micro-Circulation and Methods of Experiments" (Chief editor: GUO Yao, Ren Dong Qing, Feb. 2005).

Fig. 27 is from "Guo Lin New Qigong", TAO Bing Fu, Tong Xin Publishing House, Jul. 1999.

Fig. 7a and Fig.17 are from " Hardenberg Lexikon der Nobelpreisträger 2000".

Fig. 44, 45 are the documents of author, made by Universität Klinikum zu Köln (Jun. 2006).

REFERENCE

1. "The Basic Theory of Chinese Medicine" Chief Editor: YIN Hui He, Shanghai Science & Technology Press, Aug. Aug. 1983.

2. "The Analyze of Hepatosis cases by GUAN You Bo" ZHAO Bo Zhi, Chen Yong, People's Military Medical Press, Nov. 2010

3. "The Proven Recipes of Hepatosis by Famous and Senior Experts of TCM" XU Jiang Yan, Liu Wen Li, YANG Jian Yu, DU Lei. Zhong Yuan Peasant Publishing House, Jan. 2010.

4. "The Manual of Chinese Herbs in Clinic" Teaching and Research Section of Herbs Recipe, Shanghai TCM College Jun. 1977, Shanhhai People's Press.

5. "The Complete Volume on Practical Acupuncture" LIU Han Yin, Beijing Publishing House, Nov.1988.

6. "Famous Herb Receipt of Ancient and Modern China" XIE Fa Liang, YANG Yun Xiang, LIU Cui Rong, LI Qiong, YANG Hui Ming, He Nan Science & Technology Press, Jan. 2001.

7. "Physiologie" Deetjen, Speckmann, Urban & Fischer Press, 1999

8. "Biologie" Mörike, Betz, Mergenthaler, Nikol Verlag, 2007

9. "Neuroanatomie" Natalie Garzorz, Urban & Fischer Press, 2009

10. "Neurowissenschaft" M.F.Bear, B. W. Connors, M.A.Paradiso, A.Engel, Spektrum Akademischer Verlag, Okt. 2011.

11. "Medical Neurobiology" GUAN Xin Min, HAN Ji Sheng, People's Medical Publishing House, Feb. 2004.

12. "Essentials of Neuroscience" HAN Ji Sheng, Peking Medical University Press Jun. 1993.

13. "Medical Cytobiology" WANG Pei Lin, YANG Kang Juan, People's Medical Publishing House, Sept. 2005.

14. "Human Physiology" ZHU Shi Gong, , ZHANG Zhi Wen, Peking Medical University Press, Aug. 2002.

15. "Foundation of Micro-Circulation and Methods of Experiments" Chief editor: GUO Yao, Ren Dong Qing, Fourth Military Medical University Press, Feb. 2005.

16. "Theoritical Foundation of Plasma" HU Xi Wei, Peking University Press, Jan. 2006

17. "Plasma Physics" LI Ding, CHEN Yin Hua, MA Jin Xiu, YANG Wei Hong, Higher Education Press, Aug. 2005

18. "Calculus-Computer-Based Physics" LI Yuan Jie, LU Guo, Higher Education Press, Jul. 2004

19. "Physics of University" JIA Gui Ru, CAO Xue Cheng, China Agraculture University Press, Dec. 2009

20. "Electromagnetics" XU You, Science Publishing House, Beijing, Aug. 2008

21. "Foundation of Geophysics" SHI Ge, Peking University Press, Oct. 2002

22. "Modern Crystal Science" ZHANG Ke Cong, Science Publishing Hause, Beijing, May 2011

23. "Fundation of Acoustics" DU Gong Huan, ZHU Zhe Ming, GONG Xiu Fen, Nanking University Press, May 2012

24. "A History of Western Thought" G. Skirbekk, N. Gilje, Translators: TONG Shi Jun, YU Zhen Hua, LIU Jin, Shanghai Translation Publishing House, 2003.

25. Physiology and Cell Biology of Acupuncture observed in Calcium Signaling ctivted by Acoustic Shear Wave. Springer Open Choice, Published on 110. 1007/s00424-011-0993-7 Author: Geng Li and 13 Person.ine" 2011 Jul. 28. Doi:

26. "Systems Anatomy" Gu Xiao Song，Hu Xing Yu，Science Publishing House Jan. 2008。

27. "Neuroscience Basis" Li Ji Shuo，Higher Education Press，Jun. 2002。

28. "Cardiobiolog from Cell to Circulation" L. H. Opie ，translators: Gao Tian Xiang ，Gao Tian Li ，Science Publishing House Sep. 2001。

29. "The Mechinery Regulating Vesiele Traffic ， a Major Transport System in our Cells" J. E. Rothman, R. W. Schekmancand T. C. Südhof, 2013 Nobel Medical and Biology Prize winners.

AFTERWORD

 Since the phenomena of meridian is existence in deed, and its anatomy structure has not been discovered until now, we could try and look for explaining this fact with another way. We combine the Human Science (Biology) with the Environment Science (Solar-Earth Physical Environment mainly) to research the Meridian phenomena, based on the two scientific interdisciplinary courses. This is in keeping with the principle of " Unification between Heaven and Human" of the traditional Chinese philosophy. This is one of the aims that I write this book.

At same time I strive to build a bridge between Traditional Chinese Medicine and the West Modern Sciences (Quantum Physics and Cytomolecular Biology mainly), and illustrate the meridian phenomena with the theory of field of bio-wave. With the combination of the two sides much more new scientific subjects will be born, such as Cytomolecular Dynamics, Mechanics of Tissues of Human, Dynamics of Molecule, Relation between Bio-wave and Neurotransmitter, Electro-Chemstry and Electro-Dynamics of Cell Membrane, Reaction between Herbs and Cell Membrane, Relation between Acupuncture and Cell Macromolecule, Relation between Acupuncture and Cell Eletrolyte, Liquid Crystaliograph of Bio-Macromolecule, Liquid Crystallography of Cell Membrane, etc..

These researches all are based on dynamic model of bio-wave of living people but motionless anatomy tissue or organ of dead man. This is the pith of the foundation of meridian. This research would explore a new developing direction of physiology, pathology and pharmacology. The theory of bio-wave has been confirmed by more and more experiments. The putting forward of theory of bio-wave would develop the new way of theory of TCM and also supply beneficial thinking to West Medicine. This is the second aim of my writing.

In the time when I wrote this book, an excited and excellent experiment result announced that acupuncture induced the **transversal acoustic wave** along meridian line by Prof. Li Geng and colleagues, Hong Kong University with nuclear magnetic resonance. In this experiment they found the acoustic vibration of Transvers Wave along the Meridian, and the Ca^{++} vibration. This illustrated the theory of the "Bio-Wave of Meridian Theory" supplied by author is verified by scientific test (see Chapter 5).

The third aim of this book is to hope the scientists, institutes and universities who are concerned and interested in the research of meridian, acupuncture and Chinese Medicine could pay attention into the theory and experiment of following projects:

1. The production and detecting of bio-wave of human body;

2. The interaction between bio-wave and cellular membrane;

3. The interaction between bio-wave and cellular plasma;

4. The interaction between bio-wave and cellular nuclear

After all these projects are deeply researched and gotten correct conclusion, the Chinese Medicine could develop more rapidly in the world I think, and the West Medical Pharmacy will have a new and great way to manufacture more effective drugs and to find out better therapeutic methods.

If possible, I hope much more experts of Chinese medicine, West medicine and referential natural sciences co-operate together to research meridian in theory and practice to get grand progress. Of course, this is a huge system engineering in over century, and is the deciphering for "Goldbach's Conjecture" of TCM with 2500 years history. Just as the famous scientist Prof. QIAN Xue Sen said, "It will bring about a scientific revolution, as well as a technical revolution to change the world."

In the publishing period, Prof. Ren Dong Qing (China No.4 Military Medical University), and other people supply the experimental result and meridian pictures. Author express gratitude to them.

Author thanks for Dr. med Irene Messer who gives me direction and helps for the writing of this book.

Author

Spring 2019

Cologne, Germany

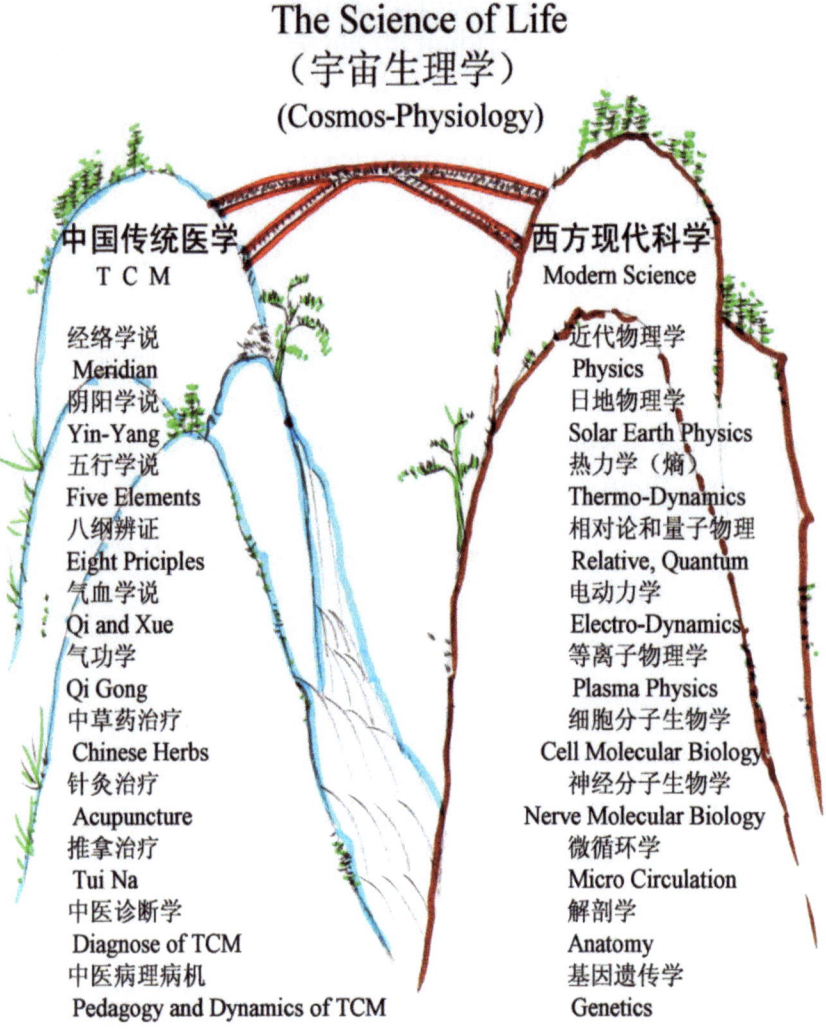

生命科学
The Science of Life
（宇宙生理学）
(Cosmos-Physiology)

中国传统医学
TCM

西方现代科学
Modern Science

经络学说
Meridian
阴阳学说
Yin-Yang
五行学说
Five Elements
八纲辨证
Eight Priciples
气血学说
Qi and Xue
气功学
Qi Gong
中草药治疗
Chinese Herbs
针灸治疗
Acupuncture
推拿治疗
Tui Na
中医诊断学
Diagnose of TCM
中医病理病机
Pedagogy and Dynamics of TCM

近代物理学
Physics
日地物理学
Solar Earth Physics
热力学（熵）
Thermo-Dynamics
相对论和量子物理
Relative, Quantum
电动力学
Electro-Dynamics
等离子物理学
Plasma Physics
细胞分子生物学
Cell Molecular Biology
神经分子生物学
Nerve Molecular Biology
微循环学
Micro Circulation
解剖学
Anatomy
基因遗传学
Genetics

Fig. 53 The Science of Life (Cosmos-Physiology)

194

AUTHOR

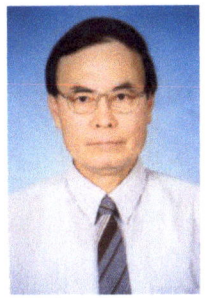

Qiang MIAO

Prof. Engineering / Physics

Prof. TCM Guest

In Dec. 1942 born in Beijing, China.

1960 graduated from Middle School of

Beijing Normal University.

1965 graduated from Tianjin BEIYANG

University, Thermo-Physics Department.

1965-1972 engaged in National Science &

Technology Commission, Beijing, China.

1972-1978 engaged in design and manufacture

of Controlled Nuclear Fusion, Physics Institute,

Chinese Academy of Science (CAS).

1979-1985 engaged in Digital Regression of

Micro-Wave Remote Sensing on Satellite,

Space Science & Technology Certre, CAS.

1986-1990 found Scientific Instrument Ltd.,

engaged in development of heart pace maker and

instruments of meridian.

1991 established THK High-Tec Corporation in

Cologne, Germany.

2008 set up Eifel TCM Ambulanz and found

Cosmos-Physiology Laboratory.

Now engaged in research of TCM and Meridian.

1986 awarded the title of Senior Engineer in CAS.

2002 appointed TCM Guest Professor in China.

2008 honored title of Professor Engineer/Physics

by Zentralstelle für auslandisches Bildungswesen

in der Bundesrepublik Deutschland.

Contribute this book to the follows respective person:

My wife Ms. Prof. WANG Li who gives me a fine and quiet environment and I could study and research with great concentration.

My parents Mr. MIAO Hong Zhang and Ms. HAN Yun Ru, who had deep loved for Chinese medicine and traditional Chinese culture, which opened and enlighted my years in childhood.

My primary school teacher, Mr. ZHANG Zong Liang in Da Shui Che Primary School, Fu Cheng Men, Beijing, thanks for his encouraging and fostering.

The teachers in Middle School of Peking Normal University, Mr. GAO Fu Zeng, Mr. TIAN Jun Mei, Ms. MAO He Ling, Mr. MI Ji Han, Mr. WANG Shu Sheng, Mr. LI Guang Jun, Mr. CHEN Ke Qi, Mr. HAN Man Lu, Mr. CAO Zhen Shan, Mr. ZHANG Ru Han, Mr. YAO Shou Nan, Ms. REN Yun Zhen, Ms. HE Ruo Qi, etc., thanks for their training with "Education of Total Moral Quality".

The professors of Tianjin BEIYANG University, Prof. LIU You Jun, Zhang Xi Jiu, WAN Xin, WAN Shi Xiong, LI Hou Sheng, YAO Biao Huan, RAO Shou Ren, WANG Shi Qing, LI Zhi Xiong, YANG Chun Rong, LI Shu Sen, SHI Ze Chang, ZHANG Mei Zhen, etc., thanks for their teaching and helping. BEIYANG University is the first modern university in China who has had deep scholarship accumulation, which makes me have the courage and capability to research and explore the multi-subjects of scientific fields.

Famous nuclear theoretical scientist PENG Huan Wu, radio telemetry and telecontrol scientist CHEN Fang Yun, Optics scientist WANG Da Hang, Physist GUAN Wei Yan and YU Lu, Prof. ZHANG Ze Xiang, who have given me the strategy guiding in my research.

Prof. ZHU Zong Xiang, Research fellow of Bio-Physics Institute of Chinese Academy of Science, who guided me to the field of meridian research.

The kind-hearted colleagues in Chinese Academy of Science and National Science & Technology Administration of China, who gave me much more helps and supervision, specially thanks for Ms. LIU Nan, Ms. TONG Wen Nian，Mr. LIU Zhao Yu. Mr. JI Bo, Mr.ZHAO Zhen Ping, Mr. DONG Yue Xian, Mr. LI De Zhong, Mr. LIN Wen Cheng, and WANG Yuan Yi etc.

版权页

德国华育出版社
出版人 李阳

Layout: Lu Han, Yicong Su

Published by
Yang Li
Verlag für chinesische Lehrmittel
www.dao-de.org